Nobody's Home

The Culture and Politics of Health Care Work

A series edited by SUZANNE GORDON AND SIOBAN NELSON

Thomas Edward Gass

NOBODY'S HOME

Candid
Reflections
of a
Nursing
Home
Aide

Foreword by *Bruce C. Vladeck*

ILR Press

An imprint of Cornell University Press

Ithaca and London

First published 2004 by Cornell University Press

Printed in the United States of America

Library of Congress Cataloging-in-Publication Data
Gass, T. (Thomas)
  Nobody's home : candid reflections of a nursing home aide / Thomas
Edward Gass, Bruce C. Vladeck.—1st ed.
    p. cm. — (Culture and politics of health care work)
  ISBN 0-8014-4243-5 (cloth : alk. paper)
    1. Home health aides. 2. Home health aides—Anecdotes. 3. Home
nursing. I. Vladeck, Bruce C. II. Title. III. Series.
  RA645.3.G376 2004
  362.16′092—dc22   2003021238

Cornell University Press strives to use environmentally responsible
suppliers and materials to the fullest extent possible in the publishing
of its books. Such materials include vegetable-based, low-VOC inks
and acid-free papers that are recycled, totally chlorine-free, or partly
composed of nonwood fibers. For further information, visit our website
at www.cornellpress.cornell.edu.

Cloth printing   10 9 8 7 6 5 4 3 2 1

In memory of Carla Neff Gordan

Contents

Foreword

For all the lofty pronouncements about the coming of the "knowledge society" and the transformation of work from manual to intellectual labor, the fastest-growing job in the United States is not computer programmer, website designer, or even telemarketer but health care aide. Entry-level positions in nursing homes or similar institutions and home care agencies (requiring no formal education and, at most, sixty hours of training, paying the minimum wage or slightly just above it, and with limited—if any—opportunities for advancement) have replaced factory labor as the portal of the labor market and have often become lifetime work for new generations of workers from the United States and abroad. As Tom Gass describes so eloquently in this brilliant book, these jobs lack almost all the attributes contemporary workers find desirable; they are poorly paid, physically demanding, emotionally exhausting, intellectually stultifying, are at the bottom of an irrationally hierarchical power structure and, quite literally, are full of shit. These positions are also absolutely essential if our aspirations to belong to a humane and civilized society are to have any substance.

While most extended American families are statistically likely to have one or more family members needing formal long-term care services in a nursing home or the patient's own home, the average citizen knows remarkably little about long-term care. The subject is complicated. It is suffused with conventional wisdom, much of it wrong. And it's something most people don't like to talk about; denial and avoidance are powerful psychological phenomena, especially in a society eager to promote the fantasy that no one really ever has to grow old. As Gass makes clear, much of the subject matter is downright unpleasant. He has provided us with an extraordinary view from the front lines, but like a journalist embedded among troops at the front, his perspective on the broader landscape is unavoidably constrained. A little bit of the bigger picture may thus be helpful.

The demographic arithmetic is simple—and belies the conventional wisdom about the demand for aides' services. Never before in human history have so many people lived so long. Most of the frail elderly who need regular help with the simple activities of daily living—eating, dressing, going to the bathroom— are cared for by family members or friends, outside the paid labor market or the ken of government programs. But a growing number of old people have simply outlived most of their families, friends, and assets, as well as their physical health and cognitive competence. Families, by and large (there are always exceptions), do not "dump" grandmas into nursing homes; if anything, the evidence suggests, they are more likely to err in heroic efforts to keep older relatives at home long beyond the point of any rational expectations. Nor do public programs still invariably push those in need of paid services into institutions; over the last two decades, there has been essentially no growth in the number of people using publicly supported nursing home care, while in-home services in the more progressive areas of the country have grown like weeds. Even the Supreme Court has directed states to treat institutionalization as a last resort. Still, each passing day increases the ranks of those who can't care for themselves and whose loved ones can't care for them—and the tidal wave of aging baby boomers has yet to show up in the system.

People of means have always employed strangers to provide intimate personal care to family members who are dependent by choice or circumstance—the Biblical Patriarchs had maidservants and slaves; bourgeois houses in nineteenth-century America had quarters for servants (in the South, the slave quarters were outside the main house); today's celebrities have personal trainers, personal chefs, and "posses." Few members of wealthy families are ever admitted to nursing homes because they can get all the services they need brought to them at home. But in this country, our antipathy to public subsidy of services to those with more modest incomes is so powerful that we provide personal care to the "deserving" poor and near-poor under only the most limited and grudging circumstances. Nursing homes were invented, from the perspective of public policy, only because continued public support of county poorhouses had become unthinkable and because policymakers thought that the availability of nursing homes would, somehow, help reduce hospital expenditures. Similarly, we have expanded public programs for in-home care slowly and fitfully, not from the impulse that it is the least a wealthy society can do to help its poorest and most dependent members but from the (accurate) belief that most people prefer to remain in their own homes as long as they can, combined with the (inaccurate) notion that home care would somehow be cheaper and better than nursing homes.

Contemporary American nursing homes are the product of such convoluted thinking. Ostensibly medical facilities, they provide very little medical care—indeed, when a resident becomes seriously ill, she is generally shipped off to a hospital. Paid for and regulated by government agencies responsible for health in-

surance and health facilities, they have been physically config-
ured to resemble mini-hospitals and shaped institutionally, as
Gass notes so articulately, by rules and regulations meant to pre-
clude the worst sorts of abuse or disaster or embarrassment, not
by an effort to create especially sensitive or responsive environments for lonely, frightened, frail old people. They are managed
clinically by nurses who have no time to do any direct nursing
but spend their days on paperwork they abhor and on organiz-
ing and supervising paraprofessionals, a demanding task for
which they have no training. And they are operated predomi-
nantly by entrepreneurs who can survive economically only by
squeezing nickels and speculating in real estate.

In this context, what is perhaps most surprising about much
of long-term care in the United States is not that it is often inad-
equate but that it works at all and sometimes works remarkably
well. And the primary reason it does work, when it does, is the
energy, dedication, compassion, and creativity of the primary
caregivers—the nursing home and home care aides, nursing as-
sistants, and personal care workers (nomenclature varies; the essential tasks do not). In general (there are always exceptions),
these workers provide a level and an extent of care far exceed-
ing what we, as a society, have any reasonable basis to expect—
given what we pay aides, how we treat them, what we think of
them, and how we fail to recognize them. Simple economic or
even sociological theory can not begin to account for the enor-
mous surplus benefit produced by these workers, who give back
so much more than they get.

As he recognizes, Gass was hardly the average nursing home
aide in background or in education, and he is undoubtedly more
self-conscious, more reflective—and more literate—than most
(one in three nursing aides has not graduated from high school).
But while he appears to be far above the norm in conscientious-
ness, he makes no claim that he was more caring or more con-

cerned with his patients' well-being than his colleagues were. He may have been unusual in those dimensions as well, but there the norm is pretty high. In his exploration of some of the emotional and spiritual dimensions of the interactions between aides and clients, Gass probably comes as close as anyone can to explaining how that can be; thrust unwittingly into the most intimate kinds of contact, human beings in radically divergent roles find some way to connect. Certainly, the experience consistently suggests that, for whatever reasons, if you took a random selection of nursing home aides from around the country and gave them a little training and some minimally adequate supervision, they would work very hard and very compassionately to care as best they could for the patients in their charge.

As a society, though, we're going to have to do a whole lot better at providing aides environments and contexts in which they can work effectively if we're going to begin to meet the challenges posed by the sheer numbers of aging baby boomers. We're going to have to provide wages, working conditions, and career opportunities good enough to attract and keep growing numbers of better-educated workers. We're going to have to restructure the workplace to more adequately recognize the capabilities of aides as motivated, functioning, adult people who make significant contributions of their own to the care process. And we're going to have to find a way to pay for their services that impoverishes neither the elderly in need of care nor their families while not presuming the impoverishment of those who work for them. Gass has provided some critical clues as to how a better system could be constructed.

In this era of continuous, reflexive tax-cutting and a public philosophy of every-man-for-himself, it's hard to be wildly optimistic about the short-term prospects of a more rational approach to the challenges of long-term care in this country. Certainly, our historical track record provides little basis for optimism, and those who would argue that our society somehow always finds a way to solve its most pressing problems ignore the last decade's experience in financing public education or universal access to health insurance. But *Nobody's Home* provides some basis for hope by demonstrating how, in the worst of circumstances, people will find ways to take care of one another. One's heart soars at the thought of the kind of caring that might be provided under the best of circumstances.

Bruce C. Vladeck

Editor's Note

As someone who has long encouraged nurses and other caregivers to write about their work, I occasionally receive a thick envelope containing a manuscript from someone who has taken my words to heart. The letters accompanying these submissions invariably stress the author's desire to help the world understand what it means to take care of sick and vulnerable human beings. Initially, I greeted these efforts with enthusiasm and hope, but now, after years of reading earnest but poorly written manuscripts, my heart tends to sink when I see another in my mailbox. When Tom Gass's self-published book arrived for consideration for our new series on the politics and culture of health care work, I therefore fully expected to be disappointed. With great reluctance, I opened the bright-yellow galley and began to read. The first sentence was a surprise—it was very good. So were the first paragraph and the first page; could this be true of the rest of the book? It was—Gass's book turned out to be a real find.

Not only is this book well written, it's also very important. I'd met nursing home aides while doing my own journalistic work. I'd observed aides in the nursing homes that sheltered my grandmother, mother-in-law, and mother before they died. I was also familiar with the literature on the problems of the nursing home industry. But I'd never seen anything like this—anything so intimate, stark, funny, and poignant.

Tom Gass takes us into the world of a nursing home in a way few other authors do; he writes this book as a nursing home aide and not as a scholar who is observing nursing home aides, a researcher who is studying the problem of nursing homes, or a journalist who is working on a story about a nursing home scandal (the kind of story most journalists write when they cover the field). Tom Gass became a nursing home aide not to study or write about the work but to do the work. Only after he started doing it did he decide to write about it. And thankfully, he has the skill to do that successfully. With that skill, Gass makes the work of caring for the frail elderly, with all its sad sights and bad smells, something we *want* to read about, not just something we need to read about. He shows us that aides and the residents they care for—even the most demented and disabled—are real, three-dimensional people. He introduces us to our country's system of human warehousing and describes how workers and those they work with overcome the obstacles that seem to systematically discourage human connection. In this way, *Nobody's Home* is a book about triumph as much as it is a book about tragedy.

In the foreword, Bruce Vladeck explains why this book is such a critical contribution to the ongoing debate about the care of the vulnerable and elderly and why it is so important to politicians and policymakers as well as to the broader public. As a member of that broader public, I'd like to inject a personal note to explain why I think the book is of particular interest to aging baby boomers such as myself. Tom Gass's book speaks to us in two ways: It speaks to us as the daughters and sons, nieces and nephews, and grandchildren of people who will—or are—ending their days in a nursing home. And it speaks to us as future residents of nursing homes, as much as most baby boomers would probably like to avoid the unpleasant realities of aging in the United States.

I first read this book about ten months after my mother had

died, at age 94, after spending over a decade in a so-called life-care community—the last two years of which she spent in its skilled nursing facility. As I read, all I could think was: I wish I would have had this when my mother was alive. Why? I would have looked at the people who took care of her in a completely different light. Reluctantly, I had to admit that I saw myself in Tom's portrait of family members who observe aides judgmentally and criticize them because they seem never to be doing enough for their parents or family members. Of course, on some level, I recognized that the aides working with my mother weren't only taking care of her, they were taking care of me. As they helped to manage her decline, they were, I knew, saving my life. If I, her only child, had to take care of her—as women did in the past—my life as a writer and editor would be halted and my life as a parent would be radically altered.

In spite of this realization, I didn't really want to know what it *meant* to take care of my mother. An aide would mention that my mother had had an "accident." Recognizing this had something to do with her adult diapers, not a hip fracture, I never inquired further. When I smelled the evidence, I didn't want to think about what it meant to toilet her, wash her, and feed her. Sometimes, I realize now, I would couch my fear and denial (of her decline and perhaps my own inevitable end) in carping complaints that I, thankfully, kept to myself. Why didn't they take better care of her, I thought. Where were they when she had to go to the bathroom? Why didn't they hook her bras together before sending them to the laundry so the hooks weren't constantly sheared and bent in the institutional machines that washed them?

What I should have asked myself was, why didn't I want to look at their work? More to the point, why didn't I ever concern myself with the conditions of that work so they could earn more and take better care of themselves—and my mother? As someone who writes about caregiving, I knew far more about the problems of nursing home aides than most of the family members of other residents. But, aside from the odd article I wrote, I never lifted a finger to align myself with efforts to reform the industry.

After my mother died, I tried to thank the aides and nurses who cared for her. I told the director of nursing that my husband and I wanted to make a generous contribution to any holiday party or staff-development fund the facility had. Could our contribution help with in-house education for staff, for comfortable chairs, anything, I wondered? No, the senior nurse said blandly, the aides were content and had everything they needed. (Really?) Send them some chocolate or a basket of fruit, she suggested. I balked at that. Here were men and women who'd spent weeks, days, months caring for my mother, and she was telling me that all I could do to thank them was give them each a piece of chocolate or a grape? So I sent them copies of the book I'd written on nursing. What I never did at the time (and have done since reading *Nobody's Home*) was send a letter to top administrators expressing my appreciation for the work of these aides and encouraging the creation of the staff-development fund that the director of nursing had said the aides didn't need. (I later learned that a social worker at the institution almost lost her job for suggesting that family members of residents in the skilled nursing facility form a "family council" to better deal with any problems that occurred there.)

That's why I feel, to use a cliché, that this book should be required reading for anyone whose family member is in a nursing home. Tom Gass had no intention of writing a political polemic in favor of whistle-blower legislation, the unionization of nursing home staff, nursing home staffing regulations, or other measures that would actually improve conditions for nursing home workers. But this book does have a take-home political message.

If we want the end of life to improve for those we love, we have to act to help the people who care for them. And if we, as baby boomers, do not want to end up in nursing homes that drive out aides like Tom Gass and his more caring colleagues, then we have to mobilize now—not in twenty or thirty years—to lobby for dramatic change in how nursing homes are run, staffed, and financed. When we've had a stroke and can't speak clearly, when we have Alzheimer's and can't think clearly, it will be too late to call our politicians to lobby for better staffing, better pay, and improved education for nursing home workers or to support other efforts that help them improve their pay and benefits and reduce the high turnover in the industry. If we want somebody to be home for us when our final address is a nursing home, we must act now to make nursing homes a better place to live and work.

Suzanne Gordon

Preface

Caution. This book contains graphic depictions of life inside a typical nursing home. Some scenes will be disturbing to adults. Health care workers are less likely to be offended. Some will be amused.

In these pages I venture beyond the pale of polite discussion to describe issues that confront us as we age. I have found that health care workers tend to be unfazed by these details while those outside the field are often appalled.

This is not a scientific field study or a clinical monologue. I am not a health policy expert, nor am I knowledgeable of the nursing home industry as a whole. What I offer here is one person's experience in a privately owned for-profit long-term-care facility located in a semirural Midwestern setting. I have disguised identities of the people involved to protect their privacy. At times I combine two or three residents into one so that their stories won't be confusing. Any resemblance of persons portrayed here to actual persons is purely coincidental.

My intention is to create a broad impression of a system through anecdotal observations. I express myself in the normal vernacular of those who live and work in this particular locale. I believe that my observations are balanced on the whole and that there is a hidden benefit in looking directly at our entire life cycle. Much of this disquieting picture is unavoidable as part of human biology in decline. Our system of care needlessly exacerbates this suffering. Degeneration is unappealing and we naturally tend to want to avoid looking at it, but there are values hidden within difficult realities.

Eventually we are all likely to be confronted by diminished health, fading beauty, and dwindling social influence and power. We should at least take a probative look at the system that is prepared to engulf our future. We may want to prepare ourselves for this challenging part of life. We may want to try to shape our future options now before we become powerless to do so. Family members of nursing home residents need to know of the daily realities that confront those who care for their loved ones. My intent in this book is to shed some light on what it is like to live and to work inside a typical nursing home.

As a staff member in one long-term care facility for three and a half years, I met a lot of good people living or working there. I began as a nurse's aide and eventually became the director of social services. I focus here on my experiences as an aide because they are by far more interesting.

Our current system does not normally bring out the best in those involved. A few people profit substantially from the current for-profit, denial-based approach to long-term care. Most do not.

Acknowledgments

I am deeply grateful to my friend Barbara Rishel. Her faith in this project sustained me and regularly surpassed my own. She kept me on track and helped me in many ways, personally and professionally.

Dr. Bradley Fisher, director of gerontology at Southwest Missouri State University, very generously gave of his time, correcting my thinking on several points. This he did despite his reservations about my political incorrectness.

Dr. Elias Chaisson, professor emeritus at St. Louis University, filled with vitality and enthusiasm, expertly guided me to impose some semblance of structure on the rather chaotic earlier version of this book.

Susan Eaton of Harvard University just may be my guardian angel. Fran Benson, Ange Romeo-Hall, Suzanne Gordon, Andrea Fleck Clardy, John LeRoy, and other professionals unknown to me at Cornell University Press dispensed abundant dignity, respect, and intelligence in the production of this book.

Nobody's Home

The Setting

The nature of things dictates that we must leave those dear to us. Everything born contains its own cessation.
—attributed to Siddhartha Gautama on his deathbed

I work as an aide in a nursing home.

Let me walk you through this little world that thrives within our sealed people-container. The economy of the building, with its flat metal roof and concrete block walls spread out low and long, is void of ambition or pretense. Like an industrial complex or self-storage unit, it is clean, efficient, and functional.

Our inventory here is medical specimens. Our product is time. We give old people a little more time. And if we lighten the burden of some family members, all the better. As long as we keep these faint hearts pumping, the Medicaid dollars and the life savings keep rolling in. With a 130 beds, my boss grosses $3 mil a year. He drives elegant cars and lives in a house that is big enough to have its own name. As a relatively well paid aide, my cut is $6.90 an hour.

I get old people up in the morning and pull clothes on them, load them in wheelchairs and spoon puree into their toothless mouths, clean them up, then put them back to bed. That's what I'm paid to do. Get 'em up, move 'em out, wash 'em off, and lay 'em down. No-nonsense caregiving in a hurry. We are the fast food of health care.

This is a long-term-care facility. Our best clients quietly stay with us indefinitely. One I'll call Barb in 308 is our newest. She's only twenty-seven, by far our youngest resident. Barb is a car-train accident victim. Her emergency surgery reworked the plate tectonics of her skull in such a way as to suggest that the doctor must have been in a hurry or just could not find all the missing pieces. Her head is permanently canted to the right at a severe angle. Her left arm is totally limp, her right arm contracted and pressed stiff against her breast. Before the accident Barb was an affectionate homebody—a moderately retarded, short, happy, obese mulatto virgin. As a result of her accident, she has become a living doll to us.

Barb never complains, never roams the halls looking for the way home, never resists her "care plan." She is a favorite here, and not just with the nursing staff. Helplessness is an endearing quality for many who settle into our line of work. Barb's eyes open and close but they do not focus. She gurgles through her trache-tube occasionally but shows no convincing signs of response or comprehension—not to me anyway.

Barb is plugged into medical maintenance. She has a humidi-fier to blow a moist breeze through a plastic tube pushed deep into her throat (this is called a "gag setup") and an electronic feeder to meter out drops of enriched milkshake directly into her belly. Another tube collects her urine in a plastic pouch hooked to her bed frame. Barb is indeed plugged in.

We roll her from side to side every two hours to prevent the onset of those flesh-eating bedsores we call decubes, short for decubitus ulcers. Intermittently, nurses move in to probe her tra-chea with a suction line to vacuum the mucusal buildup that coats the airways to her lungs. Without such clearing, Barb would gurgle and spew thick mucus from her plastic spout onto her chest with every labored breath, emitting a sputtering sound as harsh and guttural as a plumbing backup in a glue factory.

Every day we sit her up in a special chair so she can look out the window. Unfortunately the room is too small and crowded to permit her a decent view, so if Barb sees anything at all it is probably the white curtains and white ceiling tiles above the white walls. The move from bed to chair is laborious. Some nurses have us aides crank her up in a sling suspended from a hydraulic lift, which looks somewhat like a stainless steel engine puller. But most often a few of us guys save time by just cradling her in a bed sheet and hoisting her from bed to Geri-Chair (a sort of chaise longue on wheels) with one huge lead-bottomed grunt.

Many staff members love to dote on Barb. They talk to her with an intense affection and patience. They may speak to her a bit too loudly, perhaps hoping that their shouts might cut through the deep fog of her vegetative state. They stroke her arms and play with her hair. You can see that she once had beautiful hair. It's still beautiful, except for the patchwork of surgical scars and the bare spot where her skull went missing. Some ask her to blink her eyes if she understands, one blink for yes, two blinks for no. But Barb's such a tease. Perhaps she is playing hide-and-seek with us.

At any rate, when I'm in the room she just stares straight ahead. Others say they see her give various responses and excitedly report such miracles to the nurses and top staff. Thus far I've missed all of these communiqués from beyond.

Last week while I was taking her blood pressure, a speech therapist brought a kitten into Barb's room, hoping that the little bundle of fur might cheer Barb up. Barb stared straight ahead.

When a well-dressed front-office lady with painted toenails came in, she turned up a Willie Nelson tune on Barb's little boom box, snapping her fingers like castanets and dancing for Barb to cheer her up. Barb stared straight ahead.

I privately wonder whether this cheery lady would dance for

Barb if she could voice her true reactions. Does this lady have equal compassion for people who are awake and who can talk back? I have no real problem with such sweet effusiveness—it just puzzles me. I wonder what these people are seeing that I cannot. Why would they hope that Barb knows what's going on here? How could any awareness within her immobile body be preferable to the sweetness of sleep? Me, I would let her sleep.

"You cannot tell me she doesn't understand," the lady said, eager to show her upbeat sympathy. "I know she's in there." This time Barb responded by staring straight ahead. She's such a tease.

Every two hours I go in and turn Barb. I check her butt for feces, and I roll her from one side to the other. She lays clean and neat little brown Easter eggs which barely make a skid mark on her bed pad—a surprising output for a milkshake diet, but there you have it. Liquid fiber, scientifically balanced nutrition producing perfectly crafted stool. It makes me wonder if all five food groups are stacked up into microscopic pyramids within each handsome turd.

This is how I serve Barb: my body turns her body for her. I swab the strings of mucus out of her mouth and reposition her limbs. I dab up the sputum around her trache-tube. I put on and take off her hand splints to keep her hands from contracting. I strap on and take off lambskin boots to protect her from foot drop, a condition in which the ankle becomes limp. I measure her urine output. I minister in silence, moving quietly and efficiently.

Surely the real Barb is elsewhere and not trapped here with us. I hope she has found a better place. Even a dense fog would seem preferable to real comprehension. I do not seek to enhance my righteousness by ministering down to her defenselessness. I find no metaphysical use for her misfortune. Barb's condition is just a sad fact. I don't see how tending to a body in suspended ani-

mation makes me a particularly better person. She resides somewhere beyond the reach of our sweet sentimentality.

I do not seek out those who cannot snub me, as some of my
coworkers seem to do. I prefer residents who can talk back, who
like to give me some sass, or who might believe momentarily that
I am a long-lost fiancé of fifty years past. I even prefer a certain
resident who begs for attention in gushing streams of maudlin
self-pity. Self-pity usually irks me, but in this case we both know
that she is playing a game to manipulate staff. Hey, we all do
what we can.

I believe that life in general has its compensations and that beneath our infirmities we are all about the same. We are all infirm.
We all have cancer and dementia, and we are all dying. It's true
I get to go home on weekends and the residents don't, but what
freedoms did they enjoy in simpler days that I will never know?
What private realities roam free in those demented minds while
we grunts slug it out in the chaos and drudgery all around us? I
believe there may be a subtle balance at work here. Are they in
misery or are they on vacation? Appearances are deceiving. I
know what it's like to be in a state of shock, and while my inte-
rior experience was then quite sweet, the outer appearance of my
body was a real mess. In the long view, surely I am no different
and essentially no better off than the worst of these unfortunates.

Initiation

True goodness
is like water.
It goes right
to the low loathsome places,
and so finds the way.

—Lao Tzu

I am not a conventional nursing-home aide. I am not conventional in most ways. I spent five years in a Catholic seminary, which included a year of silence. Afterward I went to university and graduated with a psychology degree. I taught on an Indian reservation and served as director of a halfway house. I spent seven years in a meditation community. My interest in Eastern philosophies led me to spend an itinerant decade in Asia. When I learned my mother was dying I returned to America to care for her. The experience of attending her death process affected me. I felt that I had to perform some kind of meaningful work.

I entered this work with the vague idea that it would make me useful in some way that I had not yet discovered. When I hired on, I boldly stated that my motivation was spiritual: "I'm not particularly interested in being cheerful or sweet or polite. I just ask for permission to be real." I came hoping that I would gain some depth of character by doing good.

My sense of service came not purely out of altruism but also from a constant fear of being not good enough. I was raised by family and religion to believe there was an essential defect in my nature. So I acted as if, by bowing deeply, in humble service, thus giving myself away, I might somehow purchase my own goodness.

It took me two weeks to muster the courage to walk in the front door and actually ask for a job here.

I had never set foot in a secular nursing home before I came to work here. Previously I had viewed nursing homes as catatonic slums—Zombievilles, places where nothing happens and where the walls trap a stagnant aura of doom and despair. I thought really old people did nothing, had nothing to learn or contribute or yearn for. They just smelled like old leather and pipe tobacco, or potpourri and too much face powder. I thought nursing homes were repositories for suspended animation or the living dead. This shallow stereotype took all the life and dimension out of my elders. What I found instead was a gallery of fascinating people gathered at a pivotal point in life's journey.

Once, while walking into the dining hall after my first two or three weeks of work, I found myself thinking, "People really *need* to know what is going on in here—right in the middle of the suburbs. This place is bizarre." Of course, I had long known that nursing homes are not appealing places. But when I began to imagine what it must be like for the residents, what they must live and breathe and feel every day, the reality hit me hard. I wanted to do something more than just help the people at hand. I kept scraps of paper in my breast pocket and jotted down what I saw and heard. Gradually my notes grew into this small book.

My first days and weeks here were miserable. I wondered if I'd made a mistake, but my options were limited. Sure I wanted to do good, but I was not willing to commute more than fifteen miles to do it. This facility is just that far from home. The director of nursing (DON) at that time tried to talk me out of applying. I wanted to gag from the smell of disinfectant and urine.

Nurse Rhoda oriented me along with two undocumented Mexican applicants who failed to show up for their second day of work and remained absent thereafter. She spent an entire day of orientation talking about feces. (Rhoda now objects, claiming that she also talked about "fires, bad injections, vomit, and other disgusting stuff.")

Fresh on the floor, I felt quite slow and unpopular with my coworkers. I gagged at the pungent aroma of fresh diarrhea. I came down with an ear infection that made me want to pull half of my teeth out. I got yelled at. One nurse advised me that "perhaps you aren't cut out for this line of work." And, on the home front, my nephew teased me for working at such a low rate of pay and called me a "baby-sitter." I was embarrassed to be seen in public wearing my scrubs after work, so I kept a change of clothes in the backseat of my car just in case I had to go shopping. Shopkeepers and waitresses, seeing my scrubs, asked me if I was a doctor. I said, "No, I'm a butt-wipe in a nursing home."

But I persisted and applied myself as best I could. I reminded myself that in Tibet and Nepal there are Tantric-Buddhist monasteries headed by lamas who reserve the dirtiest toilets for themselves to clean.

Soon enough I began to look at feces as "just stuff," as undifferentiated matter, seminal, stinky peanut butter. I watched other aides scoop shit up in their gloved hands and dispose of it while talking of softball games and baby showers.

From the beginning it felt unnatural to select clothes for women to wear. What do I know of women's fashions and hairdos? Rooting through their drawers seemed off-limits. I was definitely shy about cleaning female genitals. Dirty labia seemed radically forbidden and conceivably illegal. I'd have rather kept something of womanhood hidden and even a bit sacred. I was loath to pry at their knees, opening contracted legs like a giant clam. I did not enjoy becoming thorough and clinical while spreading and scrubbing their lips. At times the smells were remarkable in their pungency. Gradually I became accustomed and then inured to these trespasses. I also became drawn in by the intimacy that followed.

I was required to take ninety hours of night classes from Rhoda. That this overtaxed woman could make a "butt-wipe class" interesting to half a dozen exhausted laborers is a true testament to her natural teaching ability. After the classes were completed we were required to pass a state-administered test at a different nursing home.

As part of the test I had to give a shower to a sweet old lady, Laura, whom I'd not met before. I introduced myself to her in the hall. We had a good time visiting for about forty-five minutes beforehand. While we were waiting our turn, I did all I could to familiarize myself with her and prepare her for what we were about to do. I was sure I had her warmed up. She was polite and cordial. But when we got her into the shower room she instantly choked. "You're not giving *me* a bath!" she stated emphatically. After a few more minutes I finally persuaded her to go along with me step by step, being very respectful of her modesty. Then just after I lifted her onto the shower chair, the examiner said, "Look down." I had her shit all over my brand new white Reeboks I was so delighted with. I wiped off the mess, changed rubber gloves and washed my hands while craning my neck around the shower wall to keep an eye on Laura. I had to carefully guard her safety. The examiner was watching. Then she shit again—more rubber gloves and washing again, then another shit. Finally I got the water on and she screamed it's too hot, then it's too cold, then too hot . . . too cold . . . too hot . . . Finally the examiner said, "Why don't you just wash her off real quick." So I handed Laura a washcloth, but in doing so I knocked the soap dispenser off the shower wall with my elbow. I fumbled to put it back up, but the plastic brackets had broken. The examiner eyed a gallon jug of shampoo on the floor, said it looked empty, and offered to get me another. She came back, I put a huge glob on a washcloth and rubbed it in Laura's hair. I said to Laura, "Boy, this shampoo sure doesn't lather very well." The examiner asked, "Did you read the label? That's body lotion." So I said, "Well Laura, let's wash the lotion out of your hair." That finished, I started drying her off. Then came more shit and more shit and more shit. I just couldn't get her clean. Finally the examiner suggested I just put a diaper on her, which I did. I dressed her and went to clip her toenails, putting on my drugstore reading glasses to see more clearly what I was doing. The rubber glove on my left hand got caught in the right hinge of my glasses but I dared not release her foot with my other hand. Pure slapstick! I finally sorted it out on the floor.

We had a good time. The examiner said that I held together very well, "considering."

Simultaneously with my rude initiation to the physical realities of being a nursing-home aide, I began to discover the residents as complete living individuals, fully co-equal humans, real people. Once I overcame the initial assault to my senses, I began to enjoy them, relax a bit, and laugh more freely. Every one of them has some kind of story to tell. The final stages of life are richly textured by trauma, endurance, and loss—character-building experiences. Sometimes, when people have nothing more to lose, they become liberated. Maybe some of that freedom rubbed off on me. Witnessing a spent life as it unravels is like staring into a campfire in the dark of night: endlessly fascinating, heartwarming, and beautiful to behold.

The Cast

There are twenty-six residents on my hall. Seventeen are incontinent. I and another aide have three hours to get them all ready for breakfast in the morning. On average, we are allowed fifteen minutes to get each resident out of bed, toileted, dressed, coifed, and wheeled or walked to breakfast. Every morning is a head-on collision against time. I am learning to be efficient and "gentle-in-a-hurry." Let me introduce you to the rest of my residents.

Skooter is a graduate of Cambridge in his late eighties. He was born in Jakarta under Dutch rule and lived for two years in a Japanese prisoner-of-war camp. He has the bearing of a true gentleman. He was a successful publisher of a trade paper, something to do with frozen dinners, I think. He is also sweet and kind. He walks with a willowy, limp-handed shuffle, always smiling and pleasant.

Skooter speaks clearly but only in response to questions and never more than one or two words at a time. Skooter is also a finger painter. He usually plays with his morning bowel movement, lightly smearing it on the bed sheets, the bed rails, and himself. Sometimes he rubs it in his eyes. Nonetheless, he carries the bearing of a gentleman, always courteous and willing to help as best he can. In the early morning, before he begins to stir, I pull a sock over each hand to keep the BM from getting imbedded under his fingernails. But Skooter prefers his freedom, and as soon as I turn my back he deftly pulls the socks off as if they were kid gloves.

Skooter's adult life has been relatively carefree. He is not nearly as difficult for us to deal with as is his Chinese wife, who did the worrying for both of them. She managed the finances, maintained a fine house, and kept the boys in line. She visits daily, impeccably dressed, continuing a life of joyless duty. I notice that she has almost no lips. Her mouth forms a straight line across an expressionless face. She is exasperated with us and complains incessantly, but she remains polite. She thinks we neglect and ignore Skooter. Apparently we never measure up to the way she would treat him, if she could. She comes in and finds perhaps that his diaper is wet or that he has to sit at his table in the dining hall for ten minutes before being served. "Much too long," she says. She does not see Skooter when he is conditioning his scalp with poop-mousse. She definitely does not see the other twenty-five residents who also need care at the same time. She knows that Skooter is messy in the morning but admits she "doesn't want to deal with that." So she complains and then the DON obligingly climbs up our butts to pacify the Mrs. The customer is always . . . paying!

I am told that family members often feel guilty about relegating their loved ones to an institution such as ours. After all, almost no one actually wants to be here. This is the refuge of last resort: a gathering of the infirm, a place to die among strangers, a temple of surrender. Some families may express their guilt by directing anger toward us, but most of our extended family members are very kind, so I am taken aback by the signs of anger or harsh judgment shown by the few exceptions.

Ninety-year-old Ro in the room next door silently and serenely minds her own business. She reads old copies of her hometown newspaper and puts herself to sleep at every opportunity. She sleeps perhaps sixteen hours a day, not an unreasonable amount in a "sleep factory" such as this. For years Ro raised minks and sold cloth by the yard in a little country town. Her husband was a mason known mainly for his craft as a decorative plasterer; her family life mostly uneventful. Like her neighbor Skooter, Ro is a quiet digger. Apparently her stool is too dry and hard for her old colon to push through her tired old plumbing. So Ro resorts to reaming out her rectum with her fingers and plopping the dark goodies on the floor, then wiping her hands on the bed sheets and frame before closing her eyes and falling back to sleep. I have never seen such stool before, so dry and hard that you could ring a bell with it. Rounded, black as coal, and very compact, it resembles a certain form of quick-cooled lava or pumice I've seen.

Nonetheless, Ro always smiles quietly, never complaining, politely biding her time. She is most happy when we are helping her lie down. Her smile is bright and toothless. She complains mildly when it's time to get up, but with a little insistence she almost invariably cooperates. I believe that her life has probably always been ruled by kindness, and that it's too late for her to turn around now. Her son says that in all his years with her, he has never once heard Ro raise her voice. Ro's mind seems logical and clear. She is very cooperative except for her one peculiarity of defecating in bed. Perhaps she's too polite to ask for help or too shy to say the word "toilet" out loud.

Ninety-two-year-old Midge used to be a wealthy and prim debutante. Now she lives just across the hall from Ro and Skooter. A glamour photo on the wall over her dresser shows her as a strikingly beautiful young lady. She is a petite yet large-breasted woman. I imagine that she was a local socialite for most of her life. She still carries herself with that bearing at times. I am told that she lived in a very fine home overlooking the river bluffs, but those glory days are now over. After dressing her one morning I started to brush her hair. "I want to make you pretty," I said. Midge looked at me with surprise and chortled, "Can you do that?"

I also put her on the potty and I wipe her bottom for her, which is not the way she remembers being treated. "Are you going to naked me?" she squawks. Her demeanor swings between the delicate and downright crude. When I ask her if she is about to have a bowel movement, she might wave a limp hand at me, in the manner of a Southern damsel dismissing a flirtatious beau, and say, "Honey, don't talk about those things." Or she might just as easily crank up her voice a full octave and demand sourly, "Aren't you going to wipe my ass?" She may also tell me in a lower, cautious tone to "be careful not to hurt my adenoids," by which she means her hemorrhoids.

Her husband, Burton, was a radio operator over Germany during the war and remained a shortwave ham until his death. He did well as a salesman for a commercial bakery out of Shreveport, then as a real estate broker, and died relatively young. On the day of his heart attack she warned him not to climb his shortwave tower, "but he lacked good judgment, so he didn't listen to me." Burton suffered his attack up there. He managed to get himself down, and an ambulance took him to the hospital. She held his hand as he died. Midge says that after Burton died she "figured God didn't care much about me, to take away what I loved more than anything."

Now she spends her days lying under a jumble of blankets and afghans, begging for candy occasionally and warning us that her head is "spinning this way and then that way and is about to spin right off." She rarely mentions Burton any more. When I greet her early in the morning, before she's fully awake, she might say softly, "I'm glad you're home, Honey." Her life is mostly morose. She is more wrinkled than any of her blankets could be and so full of sour grapes that sometimes I call her Raisin.

Recently I found her fiddling with a few coins that she had scrounged from an old purse of hers she found in the bottom of her dresser. She held about thirty cents in her palm and wanted to go shopping. Then she remembered that she had a lot more money . . . somewhere, she just didn't know where. She remembered entrusting her finances to a kind man, but what was his name? She became afraid that she was running out of money and that maybe we would "put me outside and let the bugs eat me." I wheeled her to the business office to see our financial manager, who reminded her of the kind man's name and promised that we would "never ever put her outside in any case, no matter what, ever." Reassured, Midge thanked her and said she would sleep better.

We have a physical therapist from Kenya working for us on temporary contract. He is very dark skinned. I wheeled Midge past him in the hall one morning, as he stood in his white lab coat, preoccupied with a clipboard. Midge proclaimed quite clearly, "Oh, look at the little nigger baby! He's so cute!" Fortunately, Ken was too absorbed in his charts or too gracious to show a response.

Midge muses with a giggle, "Take me to the cemetery and put me in a coffin and make me up all pretty." I can see what a stimulating thought that is for her. But more frequently she prays aloud, "Oh God, please let me die," or she whines, "Help me, help me, I'm going to die." Her lamentations test the patience of her neighbors. Marge, the surly amputee from across the hall, spits back, "Yeah, I heard them say they're going to kill you after breakfast." Shocked, Midge cries out, and Marge smirks, delighting in her cruelty.

Marge is a diabetic with a different complaint for every dull second of every endless day. She is very demanding, but she is still a favorite with quite a few of us. She is a large-framed woman with broad shoulders and coarse, burly features. A crude tattoo on her forearm reads, "Born to ?" I love her for the blunt way she speaks her mind to anyone and everyone. When I go to wake her in the morning she is always lying flat on her back in bed, naked as a jaybird. Every morning her sheets and nightgown lie crumpled up in a wad on the floor, thrown down during her nightly fits of disgust and revolt. With her wooden leg, crude manners, treachery, and surly disposition, I think Marge may be a direct descendent of Long John Silver. "If I gave my dog a bed as bad as this one, he'd a bit me," she claims.

While I'm dressing her Marge routinely chides, "I wish they'd burn that old shirt. It was worn out ten years ago." I am careful to select out any clothing that hints of feminine colors or frills. Marge, like a hobbled lumberjack, prefers dark plaid work shirts and black pants. Anything dark and brooding will do. Bright and cheery doesn't pass muster for "Old What's Her Name," as she refers to herself.

Marge likes to relate how her mother told her she was a homely baby. She laughs when she recalls her mother's words: "You were so skinny and ugly that when friends said they were coming over to visit, we hid you upstairs with Grandma."

"Mom was a nut, same as me, but one of the best women on earth. I almost didn't get married because I didn't want to leave her, but we ran off to Tennessee anyway, me and that dirt bastard. He wrote her a letter saying, 'Your daughter is in good hands,' and all that bullshit. But he turned out no good."

Marge owned a string of movie theaters from North Carolina to Kansas. She married two men, but both were "dirt bastards" and she had scant use for either.

"My first husband was a high tempered son of a bitch. One time he was mad at my new son-in-law, who was dumb enough to drive up to the house on the wrong day. My husband pulled out his pistol and put it in the boy's face and said, 'If you get out of that car you're a dead son of a bitch.'"

As she tells it, Marge and her sister bested him on one memorable summer evening. They trapped that "high-tempered son of a bitch" under the steering wheel of the car and "beat hell out of him." Then they pushed him in the ditch and drove off to get drunk at their favorite watering hole. Hours later, Marge and her sister were stopped by state troopers at a roadblock. She says, still startled, "They pointed machine guns at me." The cops said her car had been reported stolen. And then she says, "Boy was I pissed. My sister kept trying to quiet me down, but you know me, I can't keep my mouth shut for anybody." They wound up in the county jail, where the sheriff's wife happened to be a good friend of hers. Marge succeeded in convincing them that she was making payments on the car. The matter ended quickly, as did her bumpy marriage.

I've heard this story many times: Marge was a regular at the honky-tonks north of here. One night a jealous rival assaulted her at a bar. The woman accused Marge of sleeping with her husband and ripped a couple of buttons off Marge's brand-new blouse. Marge's brother saw what happened and told Marge, "If you don't beat her up, I'll beat the hell out of you!" Fisticuffs broke out. Marge's petite sister, Blondie, jumped on the woman's back and beat her on the head with a saltshaker. The fight moved out into the alley. Marge brags that in the end her opponent went home naked. "I beat the shit out of her. I was ruthless. And lots of people came up to me later to congratulate me for beating the crap out of that loudmouth." Never before have I known a woman so proud of her testosterone.

"Were you messing around with her husband?" I ask. "Naw," she says. "They were separated anyway. Besides, I only went out with him a couple of times," she admits with a sheepish smile.

Later that poor woman talked to Marge on the phone and asked her who "that big blonde woman" was, the one who had bloodied her head. "You mean that ninety-eight-pound kid sister of mine?" Marge replied. "That woman met her Waterloo when she messed with me," she concluded.

She loves to recall her best friend, Nadine. Nadine was so unruly that every landlord she had during the time she ran with Marge evicted her. "She could beat the shit out of a turd," Marge brags. "I'd yell across the creek of an evening and find out what was doing that night, then we'd go raise some kind of hell." Nadine used to tell people to go "piss up a rope and dribble down." Marge claims that they had constant run-ins with Lola, who presently lives just across the hall and down a few doors. Once Nadine told her she had found Lola's husband and son together in the Hi-Lo Theater making love in the dark. But nobody believed her. Lola's family, Marge said, was the "meanest family on earth. They used to call the cops on us every night, claiming we were making too much noise."

Somehow Marge and I connect as friends. Besides her amputated leg she has had a radical mastectomy. In the bathroom I turn her from behind, supporting her by the underarms. If I'm a little rough she might yell out, "Ahhh, you tore my tit off," just to give me a hard time. Then, a true virago, she smiles, delighted by the churlish workings of her mind.

When the thirteenth of the month fell on a Friday one summer, Marge told me she always felt wary when it comes up. "One time on a Friday the thirteenth I was at a place where we used to go dancing and a carload of drunks came by and shot up the place for no damned reason."

"Did they ever find out who did it?" I asked.

"Oh, I know who did it. One of them was my uncle. He was about my favorite uncle, too. But he was ornery. And kinda like Lawrence Welk, he's been dead for years and his kids won't bury him yet."

Then perhaps to change the subject so I won't pry too deeply, Marge asks, "What did the old maid have engraved on her tombstone?"

"I don't know, what?"

"It reads, 'Who says you can't take it with you?'"

Marge is not at all kind to her roommate, Ro. When she watches TV, Ro uses a set of headphones so as not to bother Marge. Marge, on the other hand, turns her TV up as loud as she wants, and "to hell with anyone who tries to tell her different." Marge controls the position of the curtains and the heating and cooling, totally uncaring about how these may affect Ro or anyone else. Ro demurs habitually, preferring the sweetness of sleep. Marge tells me she has "had a hell of a life," and proudly quotes her sister's deference, "You've had it your way."

As I mentioned, Marge's declared nemesis across the hall is the overly sensitive Midge, whom she loves to torment. Once, to save time, I pushed both Marge and Midge in their wheelchairs down the hall. Perhaps I should have thought about this first. They rode side by side about two feet apart. The effect was like tying two cats together by the tail and throwing them over a clothesline. Marge and Midge vied to outdo each other, shaking their fists, hurling insults back and forth, and taking mock swings at each other for the entire duration of my escort service. Both were still spitting vitriol as they entered their opposing rooms. Nothing like a good catfight to start the morning.

Midge does not take Marge's abuse well but fortunately she has a sympathetic and supportive roommate, Gracie. Gracie was a school administrator with advanced education. She had traveled the world, was baptized in Bethlehem and, she claims, was held captive by secret agents in a Stalingrad hotel for nearly a month. She is proud and happy and smiles broadly despite missing her dental retainer. She has presumably hidden it for safekeeping somewhere in the confines of her room. Or it could have gone down the toilet. She dresses herself inappropriately in odd layers of floral blue polyester prints and gray sweatshirts, hospital gowns, and black snow boots. Like several residents, Gracie is habitually packing up for a pending elopement.

Our housekeeping service supplies every bathroom with black plastic bags to dispose of soiled Depends and clothing. True to her heritage as an Eastern-European refugee, Gracie makes smart little cords by twisting these bags and binds her clothes into tidy travel bundles. Normally most of her clothes are hidden somewhere in her room, stashed in bags and boxes or tied up in pillow slips, making it difficult for me to coax her into coordinated outfits. She smiles brightly, always happy to see me and completely unable to stop talking. She talks of her brilliant life, her money, and her many family connections. "Mike Hopkins was a fine man. His affairs were all over the place. And I mean to tell you, the Hopkins, they treated me with the gravest distinction. . . . And golly, I have so very much money. More than George Westford! Much more than I know what to do with. But I keep it all very quiet, of course. You realize we are in the midst of bedlam here, and I must keep all that to myself and be very . . . ah . . . ah . . . you know, like, hiding about all that. It's so unusual around here, I don't know what to do." She never gives me a break or an easy way to dismiss myself and move on, so I have learned to interrupt her with some false excuse or to simply shrug and walk away because I have no other choice. As I walk away, I glance back and see, from her smile, that she has already forgiven my rude departure. I might also see her streaking her hair with Colgate. Hairbrush, toothbrush—the subtle difference gets lost on her.

Gracie makes her way around the building. She is at home in the head nurse's office, sitting in a wing-back leather padded chair beside a grand mahogany desk. She looks out the window and proudly waves to every passerby. She feels that she's back in her element, enjoying the sense perhaps of a recent promotion or award. Her officious display of well-being and vigorous pride delights all of us, her dominion of students and protégés.

Gracie left a note on her dresser. It read:

Winona, I spent some news pre for machine to preparing for our home to preparing for exshan machine for our real machine for our exchamadiation for our review of mechanise. I will lead to help machine. I will lead to leading much happing to our home. I so enjoy helping to send much help to sesing our sisting happening to extiting sending good expanation. I will try Winona the best she can I lead home to mail for home.

Her note reveals the trailings of higher education and perhaps some benign authority. Her good intentions are blended by a loss of language that we refer to as word salad. As this loss becomes more profound, whole words will break down into an assortment of syllables and sounds unintelligible to all the world but herself. Literal meanings of words give way to simpler truths found in tone, cadence, and facial expression. As the end nears, these lost sounds may be followed by moaning. And then silence.

Gracie takes her walker with her when she roams the halls, and sometimes, to show me how fit and happy she is, she lifts her feet off the floor by locking her elbows and holding her arms tense against the handgrips. But one morning, just as she arrived at her breakfast table, she suddenly collapsed into complete unconsciousness. She was rushed back to bed in a borrowed wheelchair. The nurses quickly checked her out and found her vitals were normal. A few minutes later, before her doctor responded to our call, Gracie came to and got herself up out of bed, apparently crawling over the bed rails, and continued talking, unaware that anything at all had happened. She had probably experienced a TIA—a transient ischemic attack, or mini-stroke. They are fairly common here. There's not much we can do about them. The diagnosis is a guess, the prescription a shrug.

Months later when Gracie was not feeling well, she notified me, "I'm so ill, I'm afraid I'm about to follow my ancestors. I wonder if my affliction can be properly understood?" Yet nothing, no affliction or circumstance can dampen her chronic cheerfulness.

Ivy is a retiring Texan of ninety-one with an exceptionally lovely head of hair, a decent wardrobe, and an unfortunately scrappy memory of dignity and independence. She hates to be helped and loathes her dependence. "I wish I had been born rich instead of good looking" is one of her favorite opening lines. When she messes in her britches, which happens just about once every three days or so, she fights tooth and nail, denying that she is soiled. Often the odor alone is sufficient to tip us off from several yards away. We find her facing the corner, slouched in her wheelchair paging through a copy of the *National Enquirer* or an old family photo album, hoping to be ignored. She denies that she is dirty, and when she loses ground on that point, she says, "Who cares anyway? Leave me alone, gosh dang it. If I ever get out of here, I'll never come back! I would have never guessed there was anything like this place in our town. Who would think such goings-on are happening right here?"

"Dirty old men," she says. She does not talk. She screams, she rants, she wails. "Why do they always send me dirty old bastards? I bet you enjoy it, don't you? *Don't* you?" She's planted a few good scratches on my neck on shower day. I let residents refuse food, but bathing is a must. So Ivy and I do get into it. She's very scrappy.

She says, "When I see my folks I'm going to preach them a sermon they never heard before, and you'd better believe it." And I do believe it.

Lola shares Ivy's room. Lola's wispy hair is slowly recovering from the ravages of chemotherapy. She keeps her head warm with a white headband or knit cap. I remember hearing a kind word from her just once or twice. She is sullen and resentful and only wants to be left alone to sleep and to eat countless packets of artificial sweetener at her assigned spot in the dining room. She is one of several residents who are easy to ignore. Lola does not ask for attention, nor, in general, does she get much of it. She rarely returns a greeting and she has no use for small talk. About the only time I've seen Lola smile at me is when I asked her if she wants to lie down. Aides are privately grateful for the recluses— those who have no desire or perhaps no ability to broadcast their concerns, who collapse in upon themselves and want only to be left alone. Their despair frees us to attend to the squeaky wheels.

Over her bed Lola has a sepia photograph of her son as a gawky teenager. In an attempt to warm up her gloomy disposition I have learned to talk about "Chas," who is now a local engineer. Lola owned a pharmacy in town for years. She signed everything over to her son when she joined our ranks. But when Medicare/Medicaid refused to pick up the cost of a medication Lola needed, we billed the son. Neither Lola nor the nursing home has heard from him since. He changed his phone and address, then disappeared. So far as we know he may now only exist in the sheltered confines of her prickly heart.

Presently we are applying a silver-sulfate treatment on her buttocks for BM burns. Apparently she was allowed to lie in her soupy diarrhea for several hours, perhaps overnight, and the acid within it seared her skin in two cherry red patches. Her bottom doesn't look so bad at the moment, but these sores can quickly open and become ghastly, one of the signs of medical neglect our hyperalert state watchdogs are attuned to.

Almost every day Lola's first words are an emphatic "Leave me alone." So I let her be for a few minutes. Eventually she yields to my insistence. "All right," she'll say, "We'll see if you have a job tomorrow." Using her last best shot on me while I am seating her fully clothed into her chair, she'll unload both barrels: "All right! I'm going to tell Dad!"

Lola gave us a little biology lesson last month. I'll get to the details directly. First let me point out that a nursing home is a repository for normal people who have become difficult to handle or difficult to look at. The likes of our residents are not seen in the pages of mail-order catalogs or TV ads. Inside a nursing home are many aspects of ordinary life grown unsightly by the onslaught of wear and tear. Consequently veils of convention and prettiness evaporate. Life becomes too real despite our best efforts to hide from it. We are more basic and more truthful here than in your prime-time yuppie suburbs. There is no hiding from the truth. Furthermore, if you live long enough in America there is a very good chance that what goes on within these walls will become your life. It is estimated that nearly half of us who live to the age of eighty-five will spend at least some time in a nursing home.

One night I had a work-inspired dream: an acrid dog turd was stuck in my front teeth and I couldn't get it out. For several days following I just could not get clean enough. I washed my hands repeatedly and disinfected them, but oddly, a scent of BM stayed with me. It was as if BM had contaminated my root memory. It followed me everywhere. I asked nurses if aides are subject to some kind of "simpatico BM" that might color the way the whole world smells. Rhoda, clinical as always, offered a logical reply. She suggested that small particles of airborne BM might be lodged in my nasal cavity. I thanked her for that comforting thought. Even when feeding residents in the dining hall during those few days, I would repeatedly smell BM everywhere. After some time, though, it passed.

BM is very meaningful to us. I know this by the great lengths we go to hide it. Who wants to admit that something rotting and stinky emanates from the very core of us? "Shit" is our most familiar expletive. We use it to attack people's pride. We eat socially, but we defecate in guarded secrecy, and carefully wipe out the trace evidence.

I don't mean to overwork this topic, but just allow me to make a point about intimacy and dirtiness in these terms: Who would you allow to clean up your anus? This thought I find excruciatingly embarrassing. The last person to perform this service for me was my mother—with whom I likely had the tightest human bond I will ever know.

I recall my daughter's first bowel movement as a moment of pride and celebration. Yet at that very moment I would have been deeply embarrassed by my own. How odd: to reject my own nature in one instant and celebrate the same aspect of nature in another. Perhaps it's because my baby was still so pure, so innocent. She had not yet learned about shame or to assume airs.

You know you are loved by someone who can smile upon your waste, but can we accept our own? It has to do with how honest we are with our secret selves.

So onward to Lola and a peek inside our own potential future. This particular episode started at about 6 A.M when I heard a med tech screaming my name, calling for help. "Come take care

of Lola," she said, her voice choked with frustration. "I've gotten her up and already I've had to change her pants five times.
She just keeps going. There's shit all over the place." The med
tech was near tears. And indeed, Lola was surrounded by a
stinky brown pool of considerable breadth. I summoned my regular helper who by then had clocked in. We noticed that Lola
was lying in liquid shit up to her shoulders. We decided to wrap
her in her bed linens and take her into the shower room to clean
her up. We gave her a quick shower, put her on the pot a couple
of times, and laid her down twice, but the brown stuff just kept
oozing out—thin, acrid, runny, and very persistent. While I was
cleaning her rectum I noticed a very hard protuberance. It felt
like a billiard ball. I summoned Rhoda, the nurse.

Rhoda donned a rubber glove, lubricated it with liquid soap,
and started feeling around inside Lola who was sitting on the pot
at the time. Lola grabbed my arm and moaned a muffled "O-o-
oh . . . o-o-oh." She jerked now and then with the pain. Rhoda
said the impaction was not the size of a billiard ball as I had suggested. It was nearer the size of a softball. She complimented
Lola, "I don't know how you are able to tolerate this pain." She
said, "It feels like it's made of gravel." She worked it with her
fingers to break it up. Then she pulled out a chunk and asked me
to put it in a paper towel. After more prodding and moaning,
Rhoda extracted her glove dripping in blood and wet shit. Then
she told Lola that it was all over. I looked at Rhoda's hand and
I could not imagine a more gruesome sight from any horror
movie. She told me to let Lola catch her breath before putting
her back to bed. Lola looked pale, but eventually we got her back
lying down. Afterward Rhoda told me that what she had removed was an entire chicken back, intact!

Lola has no teeth. So how can she eat pieces of chicken on the
bone except by swallowing them whole? A few months earlier
when Lola suffered a similar impaction, a nurse had pulled a

three-inch chicken bone from her rectum. So Lola the bone swallower was not new to us.

Many residents beg for attention. Lola repels it. Thus she became effectively invisible to us most of the time while we were greasing the squeaky wheels among us. As a quiet eating machine, she probably scarfed up a lot of abandoned food left in the dining hall over time.

What was new came a few minutes later when I found Lola lying in a three-foot circle of clotted blood and mucus. Fifteen minutes after cleaning her up, I went back to check her again. I found an equal amount of bloody discharge. We took Lola's vitals and found her blood pressure quite low. She looked even paler than before. Twenty minutes later she was riding in an ambulance on her way to the hospital.

Rhoda is an excellent nurse, but according to a newer, less seasoned RN, she endangered her license by removing Lola's impaction. Apparently Rhoda could have made herself liable to a legal suit because she conceivably could have caused a perforation in Lola's colon. Yet, if you consider Lola's great discomfort, Rhoda used common sense and did the right thing to relieve her pain. Common sense in this line of work, though, can put good people at risk. Fortunately for everyone, Lola merely suffered from a badly ruptured hemorrhoid. Normally we would have informed her family of any health-related events. But since her son had withheld all means of contact, he missed a chance to give us some grief, and Lola's family reputation for meanness was not verified at Rhoda's expense.

Joan lives alone at the moment. Not by choice, particularly. She probably couldn't care less. The truth is that Joan can be a troublesome roommate; she has sticky fingers. Joan accumulates things late at night. We suspect she has early Alzheimer's. She dresses and grooms herself adequately. During the day she sticks to herself, either stretched out on her neatly made bed or walking the halls, erect and slightly obstreperous. She carries an air of suspiciousness, and we know better than to confront her or to contradict her directly. Joan is also a passive alcoholic. Karon, a generous aide, often provides her with a single Old Milwaukee when the sun goes down. As the beer flows, Joan is prone to hiking up her britches over the equator of her belly and breaking out in song, "Sunshine, you are my sunshine. You make me happy when skies are gray." Her command of pop lyrics is impressive.

Sometimes Joan calls herself Leda. During the day she sleeps in her clothes under a quilt. There she remains poised, perfectly straight, composed, and motionless, as if she were auditioning for a coffin role in a Bela Lugosi film. When she occasionally spends an hour or two with crayons and a coloring book, she does an excellent job of staying within the lines. At night, though, she will wander about, sneaking into rooms, collecting and rearranging objects with a logic all her own. One morning I could not find any shoes for her at all. The following morning she had almost a dozen, but not a single pair. I made the mistake of confronting Joan directly when I saw her coming out of someone else's room. She drew back, feigned haughty outrage, and became verbally abusive. Then, tossing her head back, she walked off in a huff.

Zelda and her husband Harold insist on bed baths every morning. She likes to have everything just so, every doodad where it belongs, every shining blue curl perfectly in place. They have crammed the remnants of their life together into the confines of a room designed to accommodate two standard-issue beds, two boxy nightstands, vinyl chairs, and a TV. A huge storyboard layout, a patchwork of sepia photos and yellowed newspaper clippings from the society pages, depicts life in grander days. Two snapshots seem particularly telling. One records a soiree at the lake. Five young ladies including Zelda, all in frilly white long-sleeved dresses are sitting on an overturned rowboat. Prim and proper, they smile stiffly at the camera. The other photo shows a handsome young Harold with two poker buddies seated at an unvarnished table in a bar. The unpainted wall behind them is bare save for a lone calendar. Harold's fedora is turned up in front. He looks directly into the camera with a liquid grin that might seem a bit too familiar and relaxed for proper society.

Their room is far too small for all their decorative artifacts and Precious Moments knickknacks which, despite all their care and concern, assault the eye as just clutter. Many aides fight to avoid crossing the threshold into this sanctum. Zelda and Harold expect thorough service, and why not? They're paying through the nose for it. Well, actually they aren't—the state is, their wealth long ago gobbled up by unhappy investments and the cost of becoming too old. Zelda does not hesitate to ask for anything she desires. She directed me to run to Wal-Mart for Dentu-Creme, which is cheaper than the industrial-grade paste we supply from our stockroom just a few steps down the hall.

She does not hesitate to direct her favorite aides to come in early to get her up before they clock in. I cannot enter their room without having five or six extra little tasks assigned to me. Outwardly, Zelda favors me, but in spirit she seems to just barely tolerate my incompetence. Like a cat casually blocking the doorway, she has an uncanny knack for anticipating my next move. She makes this clear with her directives: "You better give Harold a drink of water before you go, dear" (she says "dear" with an astringent emphasis, as if a corset was squeezing the bile out of her gall bladder).

"Harold, drink some water! Tom, you'd better put the lid back on that water before the flies take over. I think Harold should get up for lunch, don't you?"

"Harold, do you want to get up for lunch? You ought to get up." Harold opens his eyes a slit, barely taking notice, then closes them without responding.

"Well, maybe you can get him up later. And shut the light off before you go, and close the bathroom door, will you, dear" (there's that "dear" again), "and close the outside door about two-thirds the way."

The world was made for Zelda.

She is of medium build, pear shaped, with beautifully smooth facial skin hidden behind dark winged glasses that point the way to her hearing aids. These days Zelda pulls her thinning hair back in a bun hidden under a perky wig. Her hands are twisted by arthritis, and she can no longer stand at all. Significantly, her feet never touch the floor. So she has to be lifted on and off the pot repeatedly, in and out of her easy chair whenever she wants, and in and out of bed the minute she specifies. "Where were you yesterday? I had to go to bingo without Bingo Bob." That's her lucky charm. "At about ten minutes to twelve I want to go to lunch. I hope you can be here this time." There is something about the way she is built, perhaps it is her low center of gravity, that makes her unduly difficult to lift. Or could it be my attitude?

Harold has a kind face and a massive girth. The day I met him he was prying the last molar out of his mouth with a pocketknife. Even in the best of times he moves at the speed of a creaking glacier. Lately he has developed a serious lung infection which has all but immobilized him. As a result their room has a red Isolation sign posted on the door, which directs us to don rubber gloves and masks and use red biohazard bags for separate disposal of everything that comes out of their room. We would at times spend twenty minutes dressed up in white paper space suits to help Harold sit up on his commode, just to hear him produce a single fart. All the while Zelda would be moving freely in and out of their room without ever bothering with masks or isolating herself from Harold's germs. After a short time I came to ignore those isolation games and just entered, did my business, and hoped to get out before the germ police caught me. At first I was mildly chided, but within a week all that isolation nonsense proved too troublesome for all of us. The whole idea was quietly dropped. I fault myself for having a rather cavalier attitude about infection control. I do not recall that it was ever explained to me what made these precautions necessary. At the time I felt a lot of pressure to get my assigned tasks done. Besides, it seemed as if the authorities were fixated on creating a sterile patch inside a solid mass of decay.

Demands from Harold and Zelda are somehow more difficult to accept than Marge's monotonous carping. The difference is that Zelda is polite and proper in her self-absorption, whereas Marge's style is more "in your face." She doesn't mind some lip; in fact, she thrives on it. Zelda, on the other hand, uses guilt and "formal" anger to control her world. Zelda's style says in effect, "Do what I want or *I* will suffer on account of you." Marge's method says, "Do what I say or I'll beat the tar out of you." We all know that Marge's implied threats are hollow. But Zelda's are more cutting. It is her ability to engender demeaning guilt that makes her unpopular with aides and nurses, despite her polished social graces.

Harold married above his class. Zelda's parents were wealthy. They owned coal mines and even a small railroad. They also ran a popular saloon called Halfday, named for its distance from a major produce market. Truck farmers would spend the night there and enjoy an evening of poker and beer. Harold must have been a charmer, and presumably a favored patron of the Halfday to have wooed Zelda successfully. Harold used to be a square-dance caller, and just a few months ago he would rattle off long strings of rhymes for me as I washed him in the morning. He'd ask if I could give him "a nickel's worth of five dollar bills." Months ago he had to have everything done in a specific sequence. Now he doesn't care about anything but his pain. Everything hurts. His skin is as thin as an onion peel and virtually transparent. He winces and barks at the slightest touch. Bruises and skin tears seem to appear on him almost spontaneously.

Harold is still in his right mind, but owing to his weakness we make all his choices for him. Harold wants to stay in bed and sleep, but we make him get up and sit in his La-Z-Boy twice a day. We know what's good for him. That is, we know what's good for his biology. We focus on keeping his body intact, but we don't let his protests hold much sway. We count his heartbeats while we ignore what great rivers of sentiment may course through his veins. We monitor and measure all sorts of body parts—the kinds of things that the state inspectors can check easily—but we cannot measure the man. So despite our best intentions, we leave Harold the person off the charts. All the while we sincerely presume that we are acting in his best interests. We do what we think is best to avoid censure from the state, because we can make him do whatever we want. He's at our mercy. We see his protests as just another obstacle to his care. We overpower his spirit to treat his colon, his skin, and his blood count.

Although he has no appetite whatsoever, we insist that he eat. He usually obliges, but it's clearly a burden for him. Zelda also tells him what to do. She has her own ideas of what he needs, and she lets us all know her hourly prescriptions.

Zelda would be appalled to learn how much those who serve her avoid her room. Another aide, Karon, calls Zelda's morning spritzing "her whore bath." We are clearly unfair to her. She simply insists on services she believes she deserves. At times she is a pleasant conversationalist, and she does have a sociable personality. I have heard others, who are not her aides, describe her as strong, caring, sweet, generous, and insatiable. She has a good heart, and I doubt that she notices any duplicity within herself. She is an ardent Catholic who reads her prayer book religiously every day. She wrongly believes that I count myself as a fellow Catholic, assuming that because I, too, was raised in the "one true religion" I would stay with it for eternity. I allow her to believe as she prefers. Zelda prays for us, her aides, and she praises our "good works" as a prelude to heavenly rewards.

Zelda entertains a host of visitors: Christian volunteers from the local Bible school, occasional priests and nuns, regular gadabouts from town. During the thick of her worries about Harold she chirped, a bit too lightheartedly in an almost bouncy tone, "I don't have time to be depressed. I'm too busy for that."

Months later Harold told Zelda one night as she was watching TV, "I'm sorry for a lot of things in our marriage. I wasn't the best husband."

Zelda pushed the mute button. "Oh, well, that's all behind us now," she said kindly.

Harold said, "I want to go."

"Do you think you can hold on till your birthday?" Zelda asked. "The kids are coming down from Wichita."

"I suppose," he said.

The next day as I was alone with Harold, feeding him his pureed meat and mashed potatoes, he brought the subject up again. "You just get a feeling about how long it will be. All you can do is get right with God and go on. Having nice people around you helps an awful lot. I want to thank you for that." I was touched.

I mentioned this exchange to Zelda. She pulled a switch on me. "The only one who takes good care of Harold is Gina," she said, referring to a second-shift aide.

Then she told me to pull back the curtain and straighten her bed a little better. It seems the night before there was a wrinkle in her fitted sheet and it kept her from a good night's sleep.

Zelda said to me one time, "I guess you think I'm a big nuisance."

"It depends on when you ask me," I replied.

There was a long pause. Her response was muted. I couldn't really make out what she said.

I drop hints to Zelda. I talk about all the tending and cleaning, the diarrheas and dementias, about how we can never possibly get done everything we are told must be done. My hope is that if Zelda realizes how overwhelmed we are she might get the idea that there are other people around who are equally deserving of our time. I broke it down to her this way: there are 450 minutes in a regular workday. Divide that by 26 residents and that comes out to 17.3 minutes per day we have to give to each person. Part of her knows that we are very busy, since she often ends her requests with "if you have time." Her mind knows the basic facts, but her assumptions constantly assign her much more care than we can possibly provide.

Zelda invited me to a spaghetti supper at the local Catholic Church. She offered to pay my admission. That was nice, but I declined, for I have little use for church socials. After thanking her, I explained that I am not all that comfortable in large crowds, which is somewhat true. However, I also did not want to have to explain my absence from church for the last thirty years. Zelda sounded truly disappointed. I was touched. Then she aired her anxiety about who would be around to transfer her from the wheelchair to the car and back. Perhaps, she suggested, I could drop in on that day just to make sure she got there okay.

One morning after breakfast Zelda has me wheel her down to go potty before sunning herself. On the way we pass Marge and

Marty who are invariably posted at their stakeout positions at the main intersection of our halls. Zelda waves a gnarled hand and recites sprightly, "I love you guys." Then in the bathroom we are set for our tête-à-tête. In the bathroom I become her confidante. I hear about what a terrible hag Marge is, or how disgusting Walter's cough is, or how determined she is to talk with the head nurse to get Reba fired. I let her believe I agree. Her vision is as valid as the next, and it is not my role to correct her. Perhaps I betray myself by passively agreeing with her. Nonetheless, soon I excuse myself to go make her bed or pretend to do something for Harold. I always feel a pull to move on. I am the hired help, after all.

Zelda can also be a sweet lady. She wraps her cinnamon roll in a napkin on Sunday mornings and sneaks it to me after breakfast.

Harold owned a string of small businesses. He operated a small fleet of dump trucks, front-end loaders, and rock crushers. He manufactured .22 caliber bullets. He built a small town's waterworks. Overall, these projects mostly lost money—Zelda's money. She felt her social standing slip down a notch as her financial security disappeared. She admitted once that it had never occurred to her early in life that the money might run out. Her pride may never forgive Harold for being too kind to excel in business.

Harold started out driving big rigs cross-country. He loved the freedom of traveling the open road, but Zelda would not accept such a life. She needed to have a regular home with fine appointments. Harold says that it didn't matter to him where he laid his head at night when he was driving his rig. "We just pulled over to the side of the road and went to sleep in the cabin. It didn't matter much where we were." In those days, "You never knew from one day to the next where you were going to wind up. We went all over—Colorado, California, all over." I asked him how they managed to take a bath in the dead of winter before truck stops were developed. Harold said, "We aren't supposed to tell." And he remained tight-lipped about it for some months. His loyalty to the past impressed me, but not enough to prevent me from probing intermittently. Finally, when I asked him one time, he caved in. "Well, I guess all those guys are dead now anyway. We used to carry a lot of water in the cabin—a lot of water. When we needed a bath we'd wash our feet first and then we'd put on our boots and lace them up tight at the top. Then we'd just stand naked in the snow by the side of the truck, or sometimes between trucks, and our partner would pour water over us. You weren't supposed to know that."

Harold loved to go fishing in a lazy, muddy river on a finger of land that Zelda's folks had left her. Before his current decline he told me that Zelda caught exactly one fish in her entire life. He had coaxed her to come along one day, and when she felt a tug on the line, she yanked so hard that she pitched a little sunfish up into a tree. When she saw the fish hanging from a high branch, flopping and gasping for a breath of fresh water, she immediately laid her cane pole down, went back to the car, and read a book for the rest of the day without looking up or saying a single word. Zelda does not appreciate Harold telling me this. "He is a strange man," she says. "We never talk." Then: "Harold was always a self-centered man. I'd just go along and let him have his way."

When Harold appeared to be at death's door, Zelda declined to grant him permission to go. I suggested that doing so might help him find some peace of mind, but she was afraid it would sound like she wanted him to die. So I quietly dropped the subject.

Then Harold said one day, "I want to go, but something's stopping me."

"What's stopping you?" I asked, just as a visitor was wheeling Zelda into their room.

"That," he said, nudging his chin in the direction of his wife.

Good-natured Betty saturates her bed nearly every morning. She laughs and says she will "cry me a river all the way to the sea." We put her on a bedpan, and if she can't go immediately, we give her a tickle to start her morning trickle. Or we load her onto the toilet as soon as she awakens, where she is content to half stand, then sit, and grunt and robe and disrobe for up to two hours, stuck in a mode you could call playing "dress-up."

Betty was the very first person I was ever assigned to get out of bed. As I dropped the bed rails, with a bright engaging smile Betty said, "I'm about to wet the bed." I stuck my head out in the hall and asked what I should do. Another aide advised me to put her on a bedpan. So I ran to the hopper room (where we rinse out the dirties) and retrieved one. I had never seen one of these devices before, except as a lawn ornament with flowers growing in it. I pulled Betty upright to sit on the edge of the bed, tilted her over to one side and pushed the bedpan under her, somewhere near the middle. Like many women her age, Betty has gained a lot of girth around her midsection, so I was trying to balance someone very big on something very small, and on top of unsteady bedsprings. Her toes barely touched the floor. Her arms and legs reached for circles in the air and then jerked back again to help regain her balance. Urine squirted and sprinkled the floor. Betty said with a broad and forgiving smile, "That didn't go very well." Later I learned there is a more customary supine position for using the bedpan.

Betty is delusional. Sometimes she insists that her light cord is a snake or that she's in labor with twins or that a man is hiding under her mattress.

"What's he want?" I ask.

"What does any man want?" she asks back in a friendly, knowing way, still smiling. I give her a hairbrush to smack the lurker if he rears his horny little head.

One time Betty was convinced that her son was stuck beneath her on her wheelchair seat. Frequently she believes that he is trapped in the waste pipe under her toilet.

We have installed an alarm on her chair that sounds an annoying whistle whenever she leans too far forward. She's fallen out of her chair several times in past weeks. Her wobbly legs can barely support her ample weight, and she constantly wants to change her clothes, potty herself, or play with the keepsakes in her purse. Among these treasures are a few tattered Christmas cards and pictures of her boys, Biff and Jared, when they were little tots. With the alarm installed, when she drops her keepsakes, fearing the whistle she is less likely to try to reach for them on the floor.

Betty lives with constant frustration of the heart, but her good nature still shines through. Her heart is not broken, it has just lost its focus. She only wants to find her love again, even though her husband Kent lives in town and actively cares for her. She has revealing delusions: she imagines that an adulterous woman named Wilma stole her double bed and that's why her husband is gone. Sometimes I find her crying, "because Kent is divorcing me," or because someone has stolen her children. Betty suffered brain damage, probably as a result of blunt trauma. She often talks about being beaten.

One afternoon, during a heavy thunderstorm, Betty asked me to retrieve her umbrella from atop her closet. This I did and gave it to her without a second thought as I went about stripping her bed. Moments later, there was Betty all made up with ruby lipstick and long earrings and beads wheeling herself down the hall under her bright red umbrella, pretty as a picture. Another time

Betty dressed herself in a silvery satin-polyester nightgown, put a floral wreath on her head and a plastic lei around her neck, and went to lunch proudly announcing that she was about to be married.

I passed Betty in the hall and she asked me, "Do you know if Kent is in the hospital?"

"No," I replied. Then, hoping to derail her train of thought: "I think he's singing in a rock and roll band."

"Well, I heard him say he fell and broke his arm."

"Oh, well, I guess those are just the words to a new song he was trying out."

Betty smiled broadly, "Well, I'm glad he's all right," and went on her merry way.

Betty's roommate, Paula, who is a petite seventy pounds, is terrified of Betty. Perhaps it's because Betty is big and still gets around, whereas Paula does not get around at all. Paula fantasizes a covert melodrama between the two of them. Betty remains unaware of this, being consumed by her own forlorn illusions. "That Betty is jealous," says Paula. "I like people, but not when they're jealous. Probably she's jealous of me because she's already got a husband." When I bend down to give Paula a peck on the cheek she puckers her lips and then raises her hand near her face to hide our affection from Betty. But when I get a chance I give her a nice hug and let her hold on for a few extra seconds. At these times she laughs like a schoolgirl and says, "Aw, you're a nut."

For most of her life Paula worked for a jeweler in Tulsa. She never married. She was engaged once to a man named Elmer, but his sister put the kibosh on that and Elmer apparently knuckled under.

Paula greets me with a smile and open arms in the morning.

Because she takes massive iron supplements, each morning she spews a pulsating flow of runny black BM that looks like a licorice milkshake. She's difficult to clean up because her legs are severely and permanently crossed at the hip. I was never told what happened. It's hard to peer into the creases and folds of her private area to make sure she is clean. In her embarrassment she laughs heartily and puckers to deliver a kiss, gassy with halitosis. With each new laugh comes another black spurt onto her bed pad, like used oil spewing from a punctured crankcase. To mask her embarrassment she asks when we're going to see Paris or London together. "Or can we at least go to a nice restaurant for breakfast?" I offer her a graham cracker. She says, "Aw, you're cheap!" She often mistakes the dining hall for a restaurant, where she finds the service "lousy."

Because she is so light and her legs are permanently crossed she is somewhat cumbersome to dress and transfer into her wheelchair. I often hike her up high, almost slinging her over my shoulder, and hold her there for a moment like a playful child in her father's arms. Paula looks down and laughs with complete abandon and says again, "Aw, you're a nut."

Star has suffered some kind of pulmonary embolism lately and her health appears to be fading. She is a big woman with fine gray hair tied up in a topknot. Her voice is soft and sandy, and she speaks in a tone that suggests she is at peace with the world. It's a comfort to be around her. She also has a strange dermatological condition—no one ever bothered to explain it to me—that has produced perhaps a hundred dime-sized cysts. It looks like someone has slipped bubble wrap just under her skin. Star is very independent, despite her ill-health. When she tired of the catheter that the hospital fitted in her, she just yanked it out. (Ouch!)

While Star was in a very weakened condition recently, she decided to get herself up out of bed. She made it unassisted about halfway into her blue velvet easy chair. I happened to come into her room as this move was in progress. There was Star, half-conscious, arms and legs akimbo, trying to get herself upright. Her neck was locked over one arm of her padded chair, a butt cheek was stuck on the other, and her arms, with a life all their own, were stretching and straining to get herself into place. She has implacable determination.

Recently she noticed that someone in the dining hall was wearing a dress just like one of her favorites. In fact, Star was certain it was hers. (The laundry does mix things up often enough.) She asked me who she had to talk to "to set the law on them."

I fumble with Star's hair in the morning, tying it up in a topknot that makes her look somewhat like a Japanese potentate. Star senses that I am faltering, pulling her hair almost tight enough to give her a face lift. She says with a smile, "I can imagine what that looks like." I stop her chair at the bathroom mirror on the way out. Star doesn't really care to check my work. She just smiles again and says, "It's all right." She's cool.

Four-foot-nine-inch Carla is Star's roommate. She is in good health and, thank God, takes good care of herself. The front office refers to her as a "social admission," meaning she has no pressing medical or nursing issues. (Some people enter nursing homes for the sense of safety and convenience. A few who are lonely or tired of taking responsibility for themselves can't wait to get in. But Medicaid keeps raising the standards. So social admissions are on the way out.)

Carla is neat and well polished, with all her edges rounded off. Tidiness issues from her pores, assuming she has pores. She seems well contained, professionally packaged. She keeps a diary that, I know, includes a record of her blood pressure readings, days when her bedclothes get changed, and when she gets a bath. I would hope other entries are more interesting, but it does illustrate just how narrow the focus of life in long-term care can become. On days when she is scheduled for a bath, she stations herself in the hall with a change of clothes folded neatly in hand, lest we forget her.

Currently Carla is in a tizzy over Star's health crisis. She repeatedly hits the call button to ask for a tranquilizer, "either for me or for her." Carla's concern for Star is genuine, for they are good friends. Understandably she cannot allow herself to relax while Star is clawing her way in and out of bed, half delirious. In better times Carla reads up to a book a day, mostly romantic accounts of the Old West. I loaned her a copy of a Larry Mc-Murtry novel, but she put it down and returned it directly. His blunt language disgusted her. On the very first page, Carla noted, was the word "whore." Nonetheless she teases Star, who insists that her knees be covered, for being "such a prude."

I rely on Carla's independence to grant me time to attend to those in greater need. She is a model of self-containment, compact and tidy in every sense. I might get to know her better if I had the time. But then, she just might not care about my attention. Her true feelings are well guarded.

Luna is blind and exceptionally heavy in the hips. She is still a greenhorn at being an invalid. Privately she prays, for she is very religious, but publicly she wails. The first time I went to help her get up in the morning I did not know that she was legally blind, and I offered her a cup of ice water while she was still lying in bed. A drink of fresh water helps get the morning juices flowing. Luna searched the air with flailing arms, bumped my hand, and ice water spilled all over her chest. She let me know how she felt about that with a shock wave that may have rattled the windows downtown.

Despite very poor vision Luna used to hobble down the halls with her walker, outfitted with a pink wicker bicycle basket which she had decorated with plastic daisies and loaded with daily essentials—tissues, plastic beads, and perfume. One day she took a bad fall and recovered in bed for two days. Then one of our more militant LPNs insisted we make her walk to breakfast. "If she doesn't get up now, she'll never get up." We were told to ignore Luna's protests. Luna managed to take only a few steps until her shrieks became too piercing. We could not help but take them for real pain, and I snatched an unused wheelchair for her. Later X-rays found a fracture in her pelvis.

Now she is wheelchair-bound and has a catheter and a horrendous bedsore on one foot, both courtesy of her extended stay in the hospital. The decubitus has eaten away about half of her right heel. The physical therapy department calls Luna a three-man lift because of her great weight, impaired vision, foot wound, and lack of balance coupled with a penchant for panic. But to save time I normally manage to transfer her by myself. This is ill advised, as it could be catastrophic. Luna somehow has lost her kinesthetic sense. She does not know if she is lying in bed or sitting in her chair, but she helps us all she can. At meals she cannot see food on the plate in front of her or even find her mouth with a spoon. Oddly though, she somehow manages to play bingo on Wednesday afternoons. Like many residents she has a passion for bingo. I regularly put her directly in front of a big-screen TV that she likes to watch. Recently when I quizzed her, she thought that the morning news was *Little House on the Prairie*. Luna, like most of us, is a creature of habit, and perhaps she's not watching the tube so much as just remembering, the idea of TV flickering in her mind's eye.

In the mornings, getting her up, she first asks if it is me. When I assure her it is, she replies, "Oh, bless you, hon." She's got a thing for me. Naturally I appreciate that. Every morning she stays one step ahead of me, asking for all the things she needs to feel properly dressed: her beads, her glasses, perfume, a sweater with a pocket for tissues, a lap robe.

Lately, from the moment she awakens, Luna has begun uncontrollable scratching everywhere below the waist. Her legs move up and down the sheets in a near frenzy of itching. Since she is a big woman, her compulsive actions impede getting her dressed. At least once, as I was lifting her up into her chair, she accidentally grabbed the inside of my thigh and began scratching it frantically as if it was her own.

She says, "I'd do anything for you, Tom." A few other aides tease me for my lock on her heart. I don't know exactly how this came about, but I inhale the flattery like spring air. I do not take her affection too personally, though. The general rule here: Out of sight, out of mind. Quite possibly she confuses me with someone from her distant past in rural Nebraska.

Luna is a potent spitter. I give her a swig of mouthwash on her way to breakfast. Leaning forward from the waist, her back straight and stiff, she projects a stream of fluid with deadly authority. "At one time I could hit a car outside from the schoolhouse window," she laughs.

She talks of reining in the lead horse when they were thrashing wheat on the farm near Lincoln. "I hated spiders when I was a young kid. One day I lit a match and threw it down into the thresher because I was afraid there were spiders down there. Well, naturally the straw caught on fire, so I ran to the well. We had a shallow open well with a bucket on a pulley and chain that you had to pull up by hand. So I pulled the bucket up and filled a gourd with water then ran over to the thresher to put the fire out. My mother saw me running back and forth while trying not to spill the water, so she came out to help me. We put the fire out without Dad ever knowing about it." Luna lights up when she tells this old story, or a story about filling straw mattresses, or one about feeding a green persimmon to an unwary neighbor woman with a habit of sleeping with her mouth open.

Lately we have noticed that Luna has started to speak in plurals. She'll say, "We've been having trouble with our legs itching," for example. She's also been holding a lot of highly animated conversations, ones, with a phantom partner whom she calls "Luna." One morning another aide noticed Luna apparently talking to her bathroom wall. Luna then introduced us to "another woman named Luna with her heel cut off, but I'm also named Luna and my heel is also cut off." I asked her at breakfast if she ate well. She said, "Oh, I ate half a piece of toast with jelly on it, . . . and I ate half a piece of toast with jelly on it too."

On a subsequent day I asked her if she'd like me to spread jelly on some toast for her. She said, "We eat about half a piece of toast each." My head cocked slightly as I wondered how many slices would best serve the both of her.

Melka was a fun-loving babushka before confusion and anxiety took over her life. She speaks her mind unfazed by what anyone may think. Being with her in her room is like walking into an Old World ghetto. She hangs out her laundry everywhere around her room, confuses her wastebasket with a bedpan at night, and sings Bohemian polkas. She stashes shoes, socks, purses, tissues, bras, underwear, flatware, alarm clocks, and a few odds and ends under her mattress for safekeeping. Or in her pillowcase. Or in her panties or in her bra. By morning her floor is normally littered with wads and strings of half-used toilet paper. She makes necklaces out of toilet paper, but most litter is just urine-tainted droppings from her crotch, from rummaging about her room, half-naked at best. When her hearing aid was lost for a few days, the social worker had three of us tear her room apart looking for it. Later we found it stashed in the crack of her butt. On another occasion I found about a dozen styrofoam plates stuffed in her pants. Most of her belongings are perpetually lost, victims of safekeeping. Melka herself is constantly lost. She demands to know why we are interrogating her and why her children put her here. "What is this place?" she cries. "Is this a prison?" She is subject to long and unrelenting attacks of anxiety that drive us all to distraction.

Melka seems to live in a circular labyrinth that Kafka would find perplexing. She swings between unrelenting anxiety and tranquilized stupor. She props her chin on her hand and with tear-filled eyes demands to know "the answer to just one question: What did I do? What did I do, that they all left me? Why does everyone hate me? Where are the kids? Where's my car?" Then, wagging her finger at me and squinting, she says, "You . . . *you* know why this happened!" Then I pantomime my innocence, palms raised, shoulders hunched. But nothing I can do will satisfy her angst. I start to walk away. "Yeah, sure, now just walk away," she accuses. I shake my head and lip-synch, "I'm sorry." By which I mean, "I'm out of ideas. I don't know how to console you." I am disheartened to realize how complete is the disconnect between us; we are speaking the same language while standing on different planets. She is right in front of me, yet I cannot touch her.

She is nearly deaf so I have to yell into her ear, "This is an old folks home!"

"Eight foot ten? . . . I'm eight foot ten?"

"No," I respond. "This is a nursing home!"

"This is an American home?" she queries.

"This is a nursing home!" I yell at the top of my lungs.

"Oh," she says, shrugging, "This is a nursing home?"

I nod.

"Aw," she says, now subdued. "They don't know shit from green hay."

She stands in her bathroom and scrubs her crotch like it's a washboard and occasionally walks around nude with the casual demeanor of someone who has never been embarrassed by her sex. My fellow aide, Karon, who is broad at the hips, stood beside me helping her get dressed one morning and Melka looked up and asked her, "When did you get your fat ass out of bed?" We all laughed together. No offense was taken. Melka wasn't judging her; she's just that matter-of-fact.

I got her up from her saturated bed the other morning and put her on the potty. I took off her nightgown while she was sitting there. She draped it over her wheelchair and said, "I'll save this for tomorrow."

I took it and explained, "It's wet."

"Ya," she replied, puzzled. "How come?"

Walking her to breakfast on a good morning, I might put a little bounce and rhythm in my step, which brings out Melka's snaggletooth smile, and she sings me a Slavic tune about a boy who stole a cabbage, wagging her finger at me and finishing with an infectious laugh. I wonder how much fun it would have been to befriend her a generation or two ago. She talks about baking *kolaches,* so I gave her paper and pencil and asked for her recipe. She started a list that ended with squiggles and dashes. She threw up her hands and shook her head in disgust with her own memory.

"I hope I don't have to pick corn," she says regularly, referring to three awful weeks of her Balkan childhood when she had to miss school in order to work in the fields. When we reach her table she asks for coffee. The head nurse adamantly insists that we give her one-third decaf and two-thirds hot water, because when she's jazzed up Melka can cuss a blue streak as wide as the Danube. To my taste, the coffee here is too weak in the best of times. I scan the dining hall and sneak Melka a fully loaded cup of java. Thus far I have never seen the fireworks from her which, rascal that I am, I might ignite.

Melka hungers. She often begs for food or asks, "When can we eat?" just minutes after finishing a meal. If she finds food, she's likely to stash it away. She broke into the refrigerator in the activity room recently and proceeded to eat an entire fruit salad that had been made for a large birthday party. She stuffed several tomatoes in the pockets of her sweater, then appropriated the activities assistant's jacket and put it on. She refused to yield it, innocently claiming, "My name is on it." Finally I got another jacket from her closet and persuaded her to trade.

One morning we found her across the hall, stealing her neighbor's dentures. She still has all her own teeth, but she was trying to fit the dentures over them. Another morning Melka sat in her wheelchair waiting, lined up against the wall with several others. She kept saying, "I can't shit. I can't shit. I can't shit." She usually finds a refrain and repeats it until she comes to a resolution or exhaustion. As it happened, she turned around and saw four or five other residents silently occupying wheelchairs behind hers. With a note of discovery, she said, "Oh, I suppose they can't shit either." Then she was quiet.

Melka's son, Lewis, comes visiting occasionally. He is frustrated with her and not as friendly as I would like him to be. I look for a chink in his armor to tell him how much I enjoy his mother's outlandish character despite the frustrations of her constant forgetting, but he is too busy being a tough guy. His visits become less frequent as her fears grow stronger.

Melka's roommate Mariah is a heavy lift, mostly because she is afraid the floor will abruptly rise up and smack her in the face again, as it did once before. When she sits on the edge of the bed, her short, rigid legs wave around in the air, as if she is unsure that the floor is solid. She is pleasant and usually quiet, though people say that just a year ago she used to be mobile and mean-spirited as well. Perhaps she fears that now, with only two teeth left, her protests hold no clout.

She is a modest woman unused to allowing men to see her

body, much less to clean and dress it. Mariah mumbles her objections, "Don't do that!" or "Cover me up" as I undress or bathe her. Clearly I intrude on her sense of dignity. Nonetheless, Mariah always rewards me with a kiss when our task is finished. Not long ago, Mariah suffered a serious urinary infection and we thought we were going to lose her. Now she sits in her chair, appearing to chew on her tongue, burping out an occasional chuckle. (Tongue darting, or tardive dyskinesia, is an irreversible side effect of some drugs.) Often she sings for us while stiffening her legs under the splendid orb of her belly. I admire the beauty of its symmetry, perfectly round and tight as an inflated medicine ball.

We put on a *Three Tenors in Concert* tape and turn up the volume to entice her. When she sings, she belts it out with heart and soul, like a diva sitting on a hat pin, holding nothing back.

Most of the time, though, she just sits.

Nearly every morning, across the hall in 301, Walter acts out a desperate struggle to survive the onslaught of our care. Female aides often avoid him because he hits, kicks, pinches, and bites. He's a terror for the night crew as well. Like a bilious Irish revolutionary, he shits all night long, paints the walls with it, wads it up, and throws it in the direction of his roommate's bed. Occasionally he eats it. Nonetheless, I love him dearly. He will beat on me: "What the hell you trying to do?" pounding me with his fist. The next moment, our entanglement completed, he will thank me profusely. "Thank you, thank you," intoned graciously, as if he is bowing theatrically before a large audience.

Walter used to be a high school teacher and principal in Michigan. Before that he fought in the trenches of France and Germany during the Great War. His family claims that he was just a couple of hours short of receiving his Ph.D. and that he was quite dignified, with a penchant for three-piece suits, stiff collars, and patent leather shoes. Once in his sleep he gave an orientation lecture to the freshmen tennis team. At other times he may slowly repeat a chance phrase like "I have to get up to fart." Or he may plead repeatedly for something—usually for "a proverbial beer." On his dresser are photos of a beautiful farm and of horses cavorting in the snow.

He no longer has enough strength to hurt me with his blows, but if he gets a chance, he will bite. When he is fighting me, he's deadly serious. He puts all he's got into every single attack. Something about his Norwegian accent and wild, if ineffective, assaults make me cherish him all the more. Perhaps it's the perfectly lovable way he blurts out, "Ah, bullshit." He is a beautifully crafted character, but then I admire anyone who puts their whole heart into action. Walter is a man of action.

He also knows what he wants: he wants food. And really, he's fine as long as we keep feeding him. I can see that he was a handsome man, and I envy the way his trim frame belies his unlimited appetite. He told me, "I got lost while hunting on Sunday and you people were kind enough to take me in. Thank you, thank you, thank you. Is there anything to eat, drink, chew, or smoke around here?"

Nightly Walter gets BM embedded under his fingernails, and it can be a struggle to clean them. I tell him that it's a school day or that his mother wants him to clean up for church. And likely as not, he nods a silent approval at the mention of "cleanliness," which in practice he so completely neglects. Other, more competent residents think he's vile with all his hacking and drooling, but I can see that beneath his geriatric crust there lies the heart of a polished gentleman. Vague memories of starched collars, cufflinks, and fine manners may waft up and last for all of a minute. Then, as I start to handle him, his dignity subsides and he protests, "Not so rough, goddammit." And sometimes he yanks at my heart by sternly demanding, "Treat me like a human being!"

Perhaps this hits home because I sometimes think of Walter, beneath his fading civility, as a feral animal. He can fight with fearless viciousness and then be pacified instantly with the offer of a humble graham cracker. Occasionally he remembers his dignity more clearly. Not long ago I took down his pants. "No-o-o," he objected, "I'm not putting on a peep show here. That's sinful, goddammit!" When I showed him his own dirty diaper, Walter shook his head and said, "That's not mine. The puppy did it."

Walter's roommate, Bud, was an exceptional baseball player in his teens, a shortstop in the minors after high school, and later a coach in a school in eastern Ohio. Just a few months ago he was working as the city clerk in a town of twenty thousand, so he must have been alert and responsible then. Now he is never fully awake but lives suspended somewhere between normal awareness and a coma. He is lost, I suppose, in the wraps of an incessant high-energy sugar buzz. His head never hits the pillow. It's suspended in midair throughout the night, even though his neck will relax when I manually guide it downward. He sleeps with the covers pulled well over his head, and in the morning, when the nurses have to take blood for his sugar test, he cusses and fights vigorously with the life-and-death strength of a torture victim. Often it requires three or four of us to hold him down for the two seconds it takes to get his blood sample dabbed onto the plastic card that reads his sugar level.

Bud regularly has a runny butt, and he cusses profusely whenever we move him in any way or interrupt his stupor. Clearly he does not want to be roused. He also seems easily disrupted, which probably has taught him to be terrified.

A small part of his left ear is missing, sliced cleanly off at the back to remove a small tumor. He claims that his daughter bit it off in a fit of hunger. He lets me shave him, but just barely. His skin must be hypersensitive as well. I love the ruckus he stirs when he lets out a long stream of, "No goddammit now quit . . . heifer . . . shit . . . goddammit! I told you not till Tuesday . . . goddamn . . . you asshole," until his loud profanities bring the attention of the office people who like everything to be nice and politically correct. They waltz in to express their waning patience.

I am remonstrated by our public relations lady: "Image is everything."

Right.

Bud's daughter claims that before we got our hands on him she never once heard Bud utter a single profanity. I'm not sure I believe that. She's the scorched-earth sort who blasts all her blame outward. I am told that she has difficulty accepting her father's rapid decline. She's moved Bud in and out of three different homes in eight months, blaming each of them for his decline and burning bridges along the way.

Bud can stand and he can walk perfectly well, but he cannot decide to do either of these. I have learned to trick him. I say, "Now slowly . . ." in a low drawl, as calmly as possible while I simultaneously hoist him as quickly as I can, and suddenly he finds himself afoot, none the worse for wear. He has no time to be terrified or to grab a bed rail, grit his teeth, and gird his loins against me. Of course, regulations stipulate that we must inform the residents specifically of everything we are about to do—but in this case that only gives him time to brace himself against me or grab the bed rail with a solid grip.

One of our nursing-home brochures invites potential customers to "imagine yourself in a fine resort." Come on. This is not a vacation spot. We are a business, and businesses are designed to make money. And naturally, our top staff needs to attract customers. We expect salespeople to put the best spin on facts, but we at the front know that our stock-in-trade is human misfortune. In practice we see these two realities clash every day. The foundation of this building is not just concrete. This business stands on crushed bones and human sorrow.

Regs

Regulations. We have a few. State and federal regulations loom large and heavy over our heads. By the time these guidelines come down to us they seem arcane, ambiguous, and unnecessarily adversarial. Rule is by fear of censure, by threat of fine, or by revocation of license.

I came into this work with only a vague notion of the industry's track record of abuse and neglect. But I know enough about human nature to believe that some people would starve their own parents, chain loved ones to a bed post, or worse. As a race we are capable of great atrocities, often in the name of love itself. Obviously some mechanism has to be in place to protect the helpless among us.

It is my experience that the regulations that filter down to the front lines are not always applied rationally, and that their cumulative weight adds to an already undoable list of job tasks. Everyone knows that we cannot perform all the tasks required of us in the prescribed manner, and that sometimes it is best not to apply a certain regulation, but no one is allowed to openly admit this obvious reality. Technically we are never given discretion in such matters, so in fact we are routinely in violation of what we are told we must do. We are always in a wrong position, no matter what we do. We are always coming up short.

When I deceive Bud and transfer him before he realizes what is happening, the move is accomplished in a split second. Suddenly he simply finds himself standing, for example. When I inform Bud properly, as I should, he grabs the bed rails with a viselike grip and his entire body freezes in terror. At such times it takes one aide on each side, prying his fingers loose one at a time, and a third aide to hoist him by the waist belt and complete the move. To get three aides together I must search for my partner, if I have one that day, and then walk a hundred feet or so over to another hall to recruit a willing and available aide. Now multiply this by the number of times each day that Bud may need to be toileted, changed, or bathed. (Incontinent residents must be toileted every two hours.) While all this is happening, someone on my hall is sitting in excrement, clamoring for a bath, or fighting against a bath; family members are scowling at us for our neglectful ways; Zelda wants her doilies rearranged, and on and on. You can see why I cheat, even if it puts Bud and me at some risk.

It may very well be best that a certain resident be transferred by a three-man lift—but where are the three men?

Policies devised in-house are sometimes foisted on us in the guise of state regulations. For example, we are told to honor the residents' privacy. So our beautician is not allowed to post residents' hair appointments because that would be a violation of their privacy. We put the fax machine in a locked room on a secure phone line, lest anyone see a medical request being sent or received between nurse and doctor. We cannot allow the names of residents to show on their wheelchairs for the same reason. Yet, in fact, every morning we root through their drawers while they sleep. We peer into their pants and check out their crotches and we barge in on their masturbation. Not because we lack respect, but because we must live in the real world and we absolutely lack time for patrician niceties. There is simply no other way. The fact is that nursing-home residents surrender all pride and privacy. In the end, they are left possessing nothing but their thoughts.

Our drinking water is regulated. Each resident must have a carafe of ice water next to the bed at all times. Since regulations are applied universally, it applies even to residents like Barb, who cannot even touch her bed rails much less control her call button—which, per regulation, must be clamped within reach of her immobile hands.

Residents who've had a stroke or might have some difficulty swallowing are given thickened water during meals—water, coffee, tea, or milk made gelatinous by adding cornstarch. Since strokes impair the gag reflex, we thicken fluids to make them less likely to enter the lungs. (The thickener does not alter the taste of drinks, I'm told. But I've not yet summoned the courage to lump it down.) Yet the same residents who absolutely must have thickened water at meals are issued plain ice water in their rooms. Global regulations typically seem to reach beyond common sense.

When residents complain of an ache or pain they must be offered an analgesic medication. If you feel bad, we'll put something in your body to make you feel better. And yet we wonder where our drug culture originates. "Better living through chemistry," as the ad used to say.

I understand that the long-term-care industry has earned each one of its cumbersome regulations by misdeeds and omissions. Of course, we staff members need guidelines and policies, because we are not a traditional family. We are the hired help, and just anyone hired off the street cannot be automatically trusted to keep the best interests of our elders in mind. But sometimes we are more actively distrusted: we are lumped together with potential thieves, abusers, and slackers.

But I see aides as a group of very caring people. We learn the habits of our residents as we get to know them, and naturally we tailor our dealings to fit each one. Universal directives, however, frequently impede our desire to be truly decent, kind human beings.

We are given so many directives, so many required duties, so many universally applied mandates, that it has become impossible to complete a full set of daily tasks. We are taking care of people with complex medical, emotional, and social needs. Always short of staff, we take shortcuts that put our own well-being at risk. Physical therapy might stipulate that a certain resident is a three-person lift, but as I've said, it's often more efficient to do the lift alone. I have taken this up with several of my less understanding superiors. They, of course, are pressed to insist that all our tasks be done in the manner prescribed. They have to say that. On four occasions I put forward a wager with my superiors, including the head nurse and her assistant. I bet them each two hundred dollars, which is about what I take home for a full week's work, that they could not perform all the duties expected of an aide in the required manner. I also bet them that they could not find anyone anywhere who could perform our jobs in the manner required. Thus far, no one has been willing to take my bet.

We are constitutionally in the wrong, constantly in obeisance to our overseers. A giant thumb looms over us all.

An often repeated contention is that next to nuclear fusion, long-term care is the most heavily regulated industry in America. I think it is safe to assume that our regulators are, like most people, good. They have good intentions; they want to keep long-term care under control. Their task must be perplexing. It often seems, though, that regulators are guided by political correctness and that policy makers do not understand how policies impact the direct caregiver. Regulations seem to ignore the hard realities of nursing homes and focus instead on matters that make no difference whatever to many residents. They try to legislate attitudes, not just actions, by saying in effect: Follow our blanket specifications for legally specified respect or else! For instance, we are told not to call a resident "honey" because that is considered demeaning by some. Is it the word or the motive that matters? How can intent be regulated? I ask, what does the word "honey" or any single word have to do with the content of my heart? And how many words would our overseers enter into their lexicon of forbidden terms? Fortunately, this directive is widely ignored.

Respect itself has no form. It cannot be confined to a regulatory box. It has to do with intent and context. If I were king maybe I would make it illegal for the DON to tell me, "You're nuts." But then would Paula still be allowed to playfully say, "Aw, you're a nut"?

By outlawing the words that hurt my feelings, I would also kill the words that set me free.

Back on the Hall

Rumors of scabies infestations pop up among the staff with great regularity. As I leave Bud and Walter's room I notice my arms begin to itch. Surely this is scabies simpatico. Like most people, when my attention goes to little creepy-crawlies I begin to itch, but at no specific site on the body. I just itch first here then there. During a state-sponsored in-service (lecture) on scabies, I noticed from my seat in the last row that a full third of our group was scratching by the time we were allowed to go home and bathe.

Bud and Walter both have skin eruptions that look suspiciously like the work of burrowing mites, whose scourges we have treated here twice before. Both Bud and Walter have been repeatedly treated with a potentially fatal salve called Lindane.

We treated the entire building with Lindane shortly after I started working here. Every resident had to be bathed and lathered with this potent pesticide lotion, all their clothes and personal articles bagged up, fumigated, and isolated, and all rooms strip-cleaned, before anyone could leave the halls and reenter their rooms. All of this was pushed forward in one gigantic effort guaranteed to make virtually every tenant and family member mad as hell. It takes months before lost personal articles are found again, or forgotten forever. Anything that breaks the routine here is traumatic. Many residents live only for sleep, which on scabies day we deny to everyone.

I do not know why rumors of such outbreaks are almost fancied among us aides. Something about our level of morale always has us expecting the worst of the facility. As a group we are alarmists and very melodramatic.

Jamie and Tinker are sisters sharing the same room. Jamie is forever protecting her diminutive younger sister, much to Tinker's chagrin. Tinker is under five feet tall and weighs about sixty pounds. Her voice has the tinny quality one often hears in small people. Jamie is physically more normal, but emotionally she blows everything out of proportion. Jamie owned and operated a large and successful restaurant for many years. Tinker says Jamie was popular and independent in those days. But apparently she has lost her confidence and her social graces. Jamie retains the habit of being the boss, but now no one listens.

Tinker garners the bulk of staff attention. She is much more dependent and, to many, more lovable (read cuddly) than her neurotic, insistent, and often petrified older sister. Tinker's hands are twisted by rheumatoid arthritis that sweeps her fingers off to the side like the wings of a tiny bird. Her skin looks like damp kraft paper and tears just as easily. Below the calf her legs are dark brown and purple from peripheral vascular disease (poor circulation). Her body is winding down. Or as some would say, she is circling the drain. She spends all day in bed, consumed by anxiety.

I read Tinker's medical records. In the social history section someone has typed a single word: "Unremarkable." That's quite a reduction of a whole life.

She was widowed at a young age and never remarried, so for many years she waited tables till the wee hours at a beer garden in south St. Louis and later at a bistro in Tampa. Tinker tells of a young male friend from the country who came to visit her soon after she moved to the big city. She lived in a less affluent part of south St. Louis, where prostitutes used to sit at their bay windows and tap on the glass when a potential customer walked by the red-brick row houses. Tinker's friend saw all these women hailing him and inviting him in. "Boy, this sure is a friendly place," Tinker remembers him saying. She laughs.

Mostly, though, Tinker is an unhappy camper. She spends her days with us lying in bed plotting her escape from our institution. "I've got to get out of this place, Tom. I know there's a way. I just haven't thought of it yet." She shares a few secrets with me about her emotional life, which mainly involve reactions to Jamie's interference and despair over her declining health. She talks with intelligence and wit, but she is always self-deprecating. When she loses continence, Tinker is very hesitant to push her call button because she doesn't want to bother anyone. She knows we are busy and she expresses her consideration for us by neglecting her own needs. Consequently the redness on her bottom flares then recedes, then flares up again. It refuses to heal. Her chart says she is confused and demented, but I have never seen any signs of that. Because she is so diminutive—she rides to the dining room in a child-size wheelchair—the nurses want to coddle and protect Tinker. This burns her up. She hates being so adorable.

"The hardest thing I've ever done in my life is to try to make people understand that sometimes I just don't want to eat anything. Sometimes I just can't stand the thought of food, but do you think these nurses hear what I'm saying? I'm not crazy, Tom. I know what I'm doing. But one day I almost told a nurse to take that damned spoon and stick it up her butt."

Tinker shakes her head in frustration and goes on, "I was not always a crumpled-up old lady. I don't feel eighty-one. The only thing that's changed is the way people treat me. Now they treat me old." Then she chuckles in a toothless way that says she is accustomed to injustice. People are attracted to her; in fact they dote on her. Yet she sits in her soft chair or lies in her bed, never wanting to do anything. She refuses to watch TV or listen to the radio. "It's so discouraging. There is nothing to look forward to in here. And Jamie just drives me crazy. She's always telling me what to do. I know she means well, but even the nurses are sick of her telling them I need to eat this or take that kind of pill. Sticking her nose everywhere. Nothing is ever right with her. I could just strangle her."

Once Tinker confronted Jamie for her meddling and actually blurted out, "Oh, go to hell!" She told me she felt better after saying that, and I believe her. I had noticed earlier that when Tinker sat up in her easy chair or when she sat at her dining table, her foot constantly tapped the floor in a dance of nervous energy. But following her outburst, I noticed that her foot finally came to rest.

After breakfast I stand behind her, supporting her as she walks to the toilet. She hobbles, favoring a spur in her right foot. Her bones are so small that I am afraid I might accidentally break her with my first careless move. But really, I'm hoping it is her spirit that will not break. Tinker sometimes becomes depressed and anxious, blaming herself for everything. We never mention it, but both of us know that it's unlikely she'll ever escape alive from this prison of cotton puffs and condescension. Really, it is her body that is her prison.

Tinker's eyes are bad—she is hypersensitive to light—so she avoids sunshine and wears sunglasses when she enters the brightly lit halls. Once, as I was changing her, I remarked how brazen she looked, lying on her bed with nothing on but her red-framed sunglasses. Tinker laughed and insisted I keep that image a secret between us.

When I told her that I was going to start working evenings (which meant that she would be sleeping most of the time I was at work), Tinker said she didn't like to think about that. Then apologized, "I got too attached, I'm sorry." She presumes guilt for every difficulty.

"We all have a gift," she said to me once, "and yours is being tender and gentle." The truth is that it was her own tenderness that saw the same in me. Some others see me as quite the opposite.

Selina is dying of cancer that's advancing in her hip. She is a hospice patient. Hospice is designed to give comfort to the dying. Usually it helps people die at home, so when nursing-home residents are accepted into hospice, it is a de facto admission of the shortcomings of nursing-home care. She sleeps soundly, wakes herself, and potties herself at her bedside commode, then introduces the world to either the sweet Selina or the angry Selina. Mornings favor the angry Selina, but you never know. On alternate days, she demands better service, a bigger room, a different roommate, or "a burger and fries and a fancy drink in a real glass, not no durn paper cup!" On other days she speaks of Jesus in the manner of a country-church matron and softly tells me of her overwhelming love for us all, whoever we might be.

Selina frequently complains about her roommate. She nitpicks at the lamest excuse. Fortunately the object of Selina's scorn can't hear a word of it.

Mimi, Selina's roommate, is stone deaf and just recently became incontinent. This downward slide followed a hospital visit and a new medication regime. Her speech, a guttural, raspy monotone, sounds like the squawking of a cheap megaphone. Now aides say that she is emitting a strange metallic or chemical odor that no one can seem to figure out. Mimi hears beautiful music in her head throughout the night. Often she conducts her celestial music as I sit her up on the edge of the bed. She plays peek-a-boo with her dress as I pull it over her head. She might make dancing motions with her arms or tickle my armpits as I am dressing her. Mimi is nearly always in a good mood and usually as playful as a puppy.

An outstanding exception to her euphoria occurred one day without warning. Suddenly she turned surly, threw down her clothes and fought my assistance, and cursed unintelligibly in a near yodel of desperation and anger. After some questioning, I found out that she has a single living blood relative, a niece in Kansas City. This niece, who comes perhaps once a year at best, had paid her a visit the day before. She took Mimi outside the building for an hour to smell the flowers and breathe fresh air, and then she left. The visit apparently destroyed Mimi's peace and equilibrium. Two days after the visit she forgot about the niece sufficiently to return to her normal good humor.

This makes me wonder if it might be preferable not to visit a resident at all rather than visit so rarely. Perhaps it is better to forget one's old loves and early years entirely than to rekindle doused flames. I don't know. I realize how callous this may sound, but I think visitors should either come regularly or not at all. The reason for giving should be to benefit the recipient, after all, not to satisfy one's own needs or assuage feelings of guilt. I am only suggesting that we consider the effects of our good intentions. Giving someone our attention is a powerful act.

On the flip side, a small cadre of family regulars come to spend time with residents every day. Their loyalty is an inspiration. They may come to feed a mother or sit beside a spouse, for only an hour or for much of the day, just to be with (the remnants of) the one they love. As some Buddhists say, the greatest gift you can give someone is your presence.

From time to time family members may take their loved ones out for a meal in a restaurant or for a drive down country roads. But often the confused resident becomes uneasy in short order, restless in unfamiliar territory, and soon asks to "go home now." The same distractions and variety that stimulate the young may disrupt the quiet lives of the old, who are accustomed to their lockstep routines and familiar surroundings.

Mimi uses her finger for toilet paper. When I put toilet tissue in her hand as I potty her, she wipes herself with the other hand. Her sense of sight and smell are sufficiently dull that whether she is clean or soiled, aromatic or unscented, makes no difference to her.

Lately, intermittently, something new has begun to make a difference in Mimi. She gets lost, forgets where she is, searches for a way out. She recognizes my face, questions me, "I know you. I'm a long way from home. What should I do?" I write out a response, which Mimi reads with a glance and then dismisses. I offer her a snack or lead her to her bedside, but I have no satisfying answers for her.

Generally we communicate with Mimi on a dry-erase white-board. More often, in the early morning, I wave my arms in my limited pantomime vocabulary, hoping not to disturb her room-mate Selina. If Selina hears me on the other side of the privacy curtain, she may get surly and demanding. She is rarely pleased with Mimi. I can usually turn Selina's mood around, but it takes time. Usually I simply can't take the time.

I can't take the time to help Beula from the back hall as she holds up her insistent arm, sitting in her wheelchair pulling at the hall rail inch by inch, with a long face, pleading, "Pleeeease help me." She has a way of pleading which sounds as if she has just crossed the Sahara barefoot and is about to dehydrate from lack of attention. If I do concede and help her along her way, after I have completed my little favor for her she may outflank me with a 180-degree turnabout and say coolly, "Now get the hell out of here." Neither can I take the time to help Mena, lunging forward in her chair and flagging me. "Come here, mister, I have to pee. Are you a doctor? I have to pee. Can I lay down? Will you go to bed with me?" I'm told that she's constantly feeling unsettled as a result of medication and a prolapsed uterus bulging out of her crotch. Alluding to it she says, "Look, mister, I have a ball."

As I work here longer, I come to realize that I cannot help even a quarter of the folks who plead for it.

It is not unusual to walk down a back hall and see half a dozen residents trapped in their wheelchairs, arms flailing, moaning, begging desperately for help. Nothing seems to breed impatience like a complete lack of agenda. Our residents have nothing to do but focus on their pain. At times our halls become a veritable sea of moaning, crying, begging, and whimpering. It is simply not possible to alleviate the waves of pain, anger, anxiety, boredom, despair, and loneliness. If I have learned anything from coping with this work, it is the need to say no. Before this job, I would not have thought myself capable of hearing a helpless old lady beg for my attention and keep right on walking without breaking my stride. But now I do. I do it every day. At first it's bothersome, then it becomes routine. But someone else's needs are always more pressing. I came into this work believing that I had a substantial capacity for compassion. Now, just like everyone else, I've met the limits of my emotional reserves. Under enough stress, I get short. My reserves run low. Sometimes caregivers give and give until they give out.

I slough off Gracie, hobbling down the hall in her walker, her mouth running on with the most gracious, erudite, and endless babble. I put off Zelda, who as usual assumes that I have time to visit politely, straighten her drawers, serve her momentary desires, and design her world to order. I divert Lea's attention when she catches me in the hall and wants to flirt or to bribe me to help her escape. In her dementia she knows something is not quite right; she just can't put her finger on what it might be. It really pisses her off. Words and reason elude her.

"Good morning," I say.

"That's not true," she responds.

"What is my name?" I ask her.

"Sweetheart?" she asks.

"And how can I help you?"

She objects to my unfamiliar politeness: "Well, if that's the way you want to be, then the hell with you. Maybe I'll just go shoot myself."

Gradually we all hobble, shuffle, meander, and roll into the Cedar Dining Room for breakfast. A bank of four nurses and med carts line up near the entrance just in front of the industrial-grade Rubbermaid tubs filled with cloth bibs. We are not allowed to say the word "bib." That word has been designated to be demeaning. We must call them "clothing protectors." But old people are free of such strictures and say, "Get me a bib," and we fetch one. Contrarian that I am, I call them aprons. I tell some residents we need them just in case we're having lobster for breakfast.

Nurses and Aides

It's pitiful that most professional nurses' time has so little to do with health or nurturing and too much to do with protecting the institution against litigation. Long-term care is a darling of personal injury lawyers. Nursing here is largely reduced to a cross between administering pharmaceuticals and paralegal documentation. LPNs and med techs—those who have completed a three-month course in dispensing medication—pass out pills and chart charts. RNs oversee the LPNs and med techs. One to six years of competitive education and skilled training on repair of the human body seem largely consumed by lawyer fending and pill counting. Nurses must initial the dispensing of every single pill.

There was always at least one RN on duty during the day shift. The number of nurses varied from two to three on the graveyard shift to as many as seven or eight during the day. Only one or two physicians made regular rounds among their patients. Medicaid limits payment to thirty dollars per visit, so most physicians are reluctant to accept patients in long-term care. To become cost effective, doctor visits are streamlined; doctors visit the nursing charts rather than the patients. There is also a house physician, the medical director who visits weekly. Any resident without a personal physician automatically becomes his patient. Every month a Quality Assurance meeting is held to oversee the care of patients in the skilled nursing unit. The director of nursing supervises nursing issues, the house physician oversees medical and therapy issues, and the administrator keeps the whole machine running under the watchful eye of the state. At the very basement level of this organization are the aides.

Normally it is the aides who are left to touch and nurture the residents, if the residents are to get touched at all. Aides form the front line of defense for an entire population in emotional peril. Intimacy is built into the aide's work, and loss of intimacy tears the most aching void in our residents' lives. It is up to us on the front lines to make our touch meaningful or cursory. More than anyone else in the diminished lives of residents, we can bring joy or misery. We are closer to them than anyone else on a daily basis. So our style of caring comes to represent all of humanity to them.

Unfortunately, we aides are in general recruited from society's castaways. We are often hard-luck cases, trailer dwellers who simply can't find a preferable career or, just as often, martyred do-gooders with a bottom-hugging self-validation. Typically, aides give their lives away to strangers, while they themselves drive old cars and suffer bad teeth. This job is tailor-made for putting the needs of others before one's own. Among our coworkers are many of the "walking wounded," although some of us hold our lives together rather well and are truly magnanimous and happy in this work. The need is so great for this grunt work that virtually anyone who can pass a good urine sample can probably get a job somewhere as an aide. Police records are checked before hiring. Historically though, repeat sex offenders and felons of various stripe have turned up among our great numbers. And in truth, petty theft is a constant reality in nursing homes, but such behavior by no means characterizes the typical aide. Most aides are good and decent people who would love nothing more than to work their way up into the lower middle class. And in virtually every aide and nurse who stays with us for any length of time, I have seen at least flashes of tenderness, love, and attachment. Many of us form genuine loving relationships with residents.

Emotional outbursts and blunt confrontations among staff members are, however, quite common. Staffers who come on board with a poor work ethic cause resentment among the busy bees who keep this place running. Slackers usually don't last long; some others are permanent social outsiders who draw a lot of undeserved fire. But all of us would likely do better with residents under less time pressure. Our working conditions tend to divide us.

I believe the profit motive creates a cost-cutting squeeze and this in turn causes high levels of stress. Additionally, there is the constant threat of censure by the state. Government-by-threat is truly effective if not efficient—or ideal.

Some RNs do put us down. I overheard one of our head nurses (we had three in my first twelve months here) saying, "Aides are a lower caliber of people." And, as demoralizing as it sounds, I do know the truth she speaks of, at least in my own life. Maybe I should have been offended, but I wasn't, not really. This is a low-class job, but that does not mean it has no moral value. Someone said, "We tell the world what we are worth, and the world takes us at our word." I found that a lot of med techs seem to have enhanced regard for the pecking order, even though they have little pecking power. Administrators officially try to prop us up at our in-service meetings, but the daily realities of ubiquitous fecal fumes, solicitous and demanding patients, and low pay cement our place in the grand scheme of things. A fragile sense of self-worth seems to be a virtual prerequisite to being drawn to our work.

We staff members administer health care, but as a group we ourselves are not healthy people. We do not even have a clear idea of what health is, beyond the obvious: when you're sick you don't have it.

By my count, more than 60 percent of us at this facility are smokers (about one quarter of adult Americans smoke). A few of us are morbidly obese. It appears that we health care workers cope with stress by putting things into our mouths. As a culture we Americans associate food (or tobacco, etc.) with nurturance. A mother is often hurt if her Thanksgiving guests stop eating the turkey and dressing before they have stretched their bellies to the point of discomfort. As a kid I was proud of how many pancakes I could pack down my gullet at a single sitting.

Our nursing homes illustrate the final outcome of such misguided indulgences. In effect our actions say, "Are you lonely? Here, have some ice cream." Conventional wisdom says that we are all too ready to stuff ourselves because of a yearning we wish to fill within our own lives. I know I overeat at times out of boredom and loneliness. Food can be a destructive habit.

I respect the complex motivations that bring each of us to a caring profession. I don't want to judge paid caregivers too harshly. After all, I am one. Self-help professionals might well consider the lot of us codependents. So often we foist our good deeds onto the helpless, whether they need it or not. We simply cannot *not* give.

There must be something wrong in our collective thinking that we caregivers care for ourselves so poorly. It also reflects a weakness in our conventional health care model.

We call ourselves health care workers.

Health: we're not talking here about "health" in "health spa," "health nut," "healthy living," or "healthy diet." When I ask my coworkers what health is they regularly define it in terms of illness. Rhoda, who is brilliant, quickly responds, "Health is lack of disease."

We are a clinical lot. We strive to create a hospital-like aura here. We wear scrubs and we mobilize ourselves to kill germs fast.

With all due respect to Rhoda and her education, let us reflect for a second. If you can recall a time in the past when you were feeling really great—you'd just fallen in love, landed a good job, won a difficult race, earned a degree—and you remember what that felt like, it is clearly something more than just "not feeling sick." When children romp and race in the backyard, they're not saying, "Oh boy, I don't have a headache!" They are fully occupied with feeling wonderful and happy, as a positive known quality. Health and wholeness may be fleeting, elusive, and impossible to quantify, but they are real.

These are the symptoms of health, but since we can't measure wholeness, boundless expansion, peak experiences, or contentment, we simply act as though they don't exist. We health care workers literally put true health out of our mind. We absolutely discount it as a positive reality, or we count it as a form of sickness: for example, mania.

I doubt that good marriage counselors define success like this: "When you two stop pummeling each other, you'll have a healthy marriage." We are allowed to get a little loftier than that.

If Jesus were in our health care system today, we would miss the content of his message. We'd be too busy treating his messiah complex. Thinking about health as the absence of disease is as helpful as defining light as the absence of darkness. Or try to build a theology out of this notion: Remove all the evil from the devil and what you have left is God. What kind of heavy and cumbersome religion could come out of that? Our current sense of health effectively contends that only sickness matters (because only sickness pays).

People go to a hospital to get fixed up and then return home. But people generally go to a nursing home fully expecting to get worse and die. I suggest that we could more accurately call ourselves "sick care workers," "diseasers," or "infirmers," for it is illness and infirmity that are our real employers. Ill health directs our actions, charts our success, and guarantees our paychecks. We man a staging area for death. This is a holding cell for the more merciful angels of our morbidity. For some, this place is Numb Pharmacy.

Our administrator refuses to call this a nursing home. "It's not a home. This is a nursing facility," she insists, thus setting the clinical tone for the rest of us to follow.

Lot's Wife

I rush to pour coffee or feed Marty if she is crying. She reclines in her Geri-Chair, which she always keeps in the most reclined position.

I forgot to formally introduce you to Marty in the regular lineup of hall residents. She'll threaten to kill me when she finds out that I neglected her up to this point. We are friends. Marty is Barb's roommate in 308. She's blessed with youthful skin and a clear mind. She also has hooked claws where her fingers used to be. They were made useless by muscle contractions from advancing Parkinson's disease. She can neither stand nor operate her arms. Her fingers are locked in extremely tight angles and her legs are pulling up and gradually fusing her into a fetal position. She can raise her arms a bit at the shoulders and she can move one thumb. Her emotions are very frail—she cries like a baby at the simplest frustration—but her mind and her humor are usually clear. She carries on normal conversations, recites poetry, and makes sharp, if cynical, observations about the staff and her cohabitants.

"I always wanted to be a poet. Or maybe to invent something," she says.

"Like what kind of thing did you want to invent?" I ask.

"I wanted to invent the electric mixer," she jibes with an acerbic smile.

Marty will call me as soon as I come within earshot and ask, "Tom, does my son still live at Indian Lake?" I assure her that he does. Like Lot's wife, Marty cannot resist looking back.

I am not her only gofer; she will call on anyone at all who is willing to respond. Then, belying her intelligence, she will ask, "When's Sunday?" referring to the day her son comes to visit. Then we will count off the days remaining. If time would allow it, this conversation could go on endlessly. It is not really a conversation. Marty, with her constant and insatiable need to be comforted, is just begging for reassurance. She is petrified that her son will not show up and love will abandon her. "I just want to make sure," she says. For sixteen years her son has cared for her and her disease. He comes like clockwork twice a week. He brings candy and small gifts and stays by her side for an hour or two, at the start of which Marty typically cries for a short while. They share conversations with other visiting caregivers. Sometimes Marty sleeps through these visits.

Her son's name is Bert. He was a jet pilot over Vietnam. "The sport of kings," he reports with a broad smile and bright eyes. In my mind, Bert is a hero at least twice over. I cannot plumb the depths of his loyalty. Now he's bald and just about deaf. He runs a hobby farm alone and cares for Marty, but she has become more than enough to handle for a single man who is himself in perilous health. This summer Bert drove out West and was gone for a couple of weeks. When he sent a card from Yosemite, jealous Marty said, "I hope a bear eats him."

Marty will call me from a considerable distance to ask the same inane questions over and over and over again. Time and again I plod my way over to her side and respond to her plea. She literally lives from one of Bert's visits to the next. He comes every Sunday and Wednesday. Even five minutes after he is gone, she will begin gnawing at us again, "Does my son still live at Indian Lake? How many days till Wednesday?" Or she may philosophize, "Who decides what day it is?"

When I get her up in the morning, I roll her to one side to wipe clean her bottom and I always slap her on the butt. It makes her smile. She's so afraid of becoming ugly and unloved. Yet it is happening.

I saw a young woman visit Marty. She had not seen Marty in years, so she was not prepared for the change in Marty's appearance. Her visit was brief, cut short by a rush of pity. She ran out of the building, bawling uncontrollably.

Marty craves attention, and when I am feeding her in the dining hall, she has all of it. I touch her arm or lightly massage the stone-hard ligaments under her contracted knees. I understand that we all need touch. I hope to loosen her spring-steel rigidity. For a while I even hoped I might have a lasting effect on her. I thought I might be able to ease her pain. She suspects that I am coming on to her and thus feels flattered.

The other day I told her how David, a rather handsome and younger resident with early Alzheimer's, managed to slip his tongue into the mouth of my fellow aide Karon. He took her by surprise while she was tending to him quite closely. Marty's response was, "I've never been French-kissed." I was stunned by sadness for her. I had no response.

Marty hangs on to my attention by chewing her food hundreds of times before swallowing. While drinking she caps the end of her straw with the tip of her tongue, just to delay my departure. Occasionally I make a countermove: I get up unannounced and feed Naomi or Luna for awhile.

If I am gone feeding others too long, she may slide into her trance, her head gradually listing forty-five degrees to the right, her right elbow hyperextended. Her slip into oblivion tells me that she is no longer available for conversation or for tests of will.

Her mouth drops, her eyes glaze, and she falls into a stupor for a few hours. I roll her Geri-Chair out to the head of the hall.

Every day she and Marge spend their mornings together at a strategic vantage point at the front nurses' station, where three halls converge near the entrance to the dining hall. They sit watching and trading comments about how our nursing home really operates.

Feeding

I am not a particularly good feeder. Some aides like feeding residents because mealtime is "kick back" time. You get to sit down, spoon-feed residents, and chat with fellow aides. Most aides take a load off their feet and converse with each other at these times. This is understandable, since the majority of residents who need to be fed are silent or make impish squeals or birdcalls while waiting for the next spoonful of predigested nourishment. Aides tend to talk across tables to each other, since most residents can't participate in conversations.

Time so transforms a body that we often forget that there is still a real person hiding behind all those wrinkles and thick glasses. This is especially true when the connection is lost—when the body forgets how to speak our lingo, or when it just stops feigning interest in our mundane affairs: a boyfriend's shenanigans, NASCAR races, or the bridal shower last Saturday.

I can do without this dalliance; I prefer to keep moving. I bounce from one table to another, priming one slack-jawed resident with a spoonful of grub, then moving on to the next. I also find some other task for myself, such as ferrying residents when they beg to be pottied or put to bed. Feeding regimes somehow disquiet me. Many residents will stare off in space and by reflex continue to open their mouths for as long as you offer to feed them. We urge them to eat, and they oblige. It may not occur to them to stop. Some lack a sense of satiety or hunger; some forget what food is. Many reach their own level of satiety, which often falls short of our nutritional goals for them. Some nurses and aides insist that recalcitrant residents eat all their food before returning to their rooms. Hungry or not, like it or lump it, they must clean their plates. I ate under the same orders when I was a child.

Maud, for instance, was once a champion stock car driver; the first woman allowed to drive in some county fair in Colorado. While driving a few years ago (at the age of seventy-nine!) she rounded a blind corner too fast and careened her red Camaro into a tree. As a result she's wheelchair bound, catheterized, near toothless, and without appetite. I can understand that she wouldn't want to eat.

One day Ro pleaded with me to allow her to stay in bed. "I don't feel good; can't you bring me something here?" So I ordered a room tray for her. Upon getting wind of this, her nurse stomped down the hall. Fuming at my insolence, she made Ro get up and forced her to eat breakfast. Apparently I had crossed the line and usurped a decision of a higher pay scale. Some people might suspect a control issue here. I guess the nurse was angry with me but took it out on Ro. If you can't meet your needs in the adult world, at least you can find a satisfying sense of control over the infirm.

Many times I have seen little acts that in effect say, "I am the only one who can do X satisfactorily. Here, let me negate what you just did." And as low man on the totem pole, I don't mind being overridden. I am out of my element here, so I step back and let them be. I need to get along a lot more than I need to be right.

I find myself in a society of infirm women governed by inscrutable women. Men, thank God, die early. This home is of women, for women, and run by women. In other words, most of the time I don't have a clue as to what's really going on here.

Nonetheless, I can't help wondering what Ro might be experiencing. When she says she has no appetite, how do we know that she is talking out of her mind? Why don't her words count? Could it be because she lacks the power to act on them? Sooner or later just about all of us become social nonentities.

Harold eats in his room. When I am feeding him and he says no two or three times, I set the food aside. Another meal will come along soon enough. Harold is mentally competent and he is paying good money to be cared for. Other aides and nurses get far more food down his gullet than I do, and they see that as an accomplishment. Perhaps. We'd like to see him with a healthy appetite, like when he was fifteen years old working in the fields, bragging about how many pancakes he could eat. That would be great. It would be great, too, if his mother was still cooking for him, measuring her love through an abundance of calories.

Gilda is at least fifty pounds overweight. She likes to drink milk, but we hold it back from her until she cleans her plate, "or else she'll just fill up on milk." If she were allowed to have her milk, maybe she would feel a tiny bit more in control of her life. She might even lose a few pounds and consequently feel better. Most people like the feeling of having lost weight. Certainly she would be easier to lift on and off the potty, which might mean she would be avoided less frequently by the aides, but I am certain the nutritionist has a more educated opinion.

Everyone here seems afraid of weight loss. I understand that people have actually starved to death in nursing homes, but given the low cost of food in America, I suspect they are rare. Our nursing home spends $3.25 per resident per day on food. Carbohydrates are cheap. This is the land of plenty, and certainly no nursing-home resident needs to go hungry. But I see no need for force-feeding, which can be invasive and insensitive. Obesity is not seen as a problem, but when a resident loses weight the facility takes it as threatening to its mission, as if not being overstuffed with calories were clear evidence of neglect. This is not our fault entirely. The state mandates that residents not lose more than 5 percent of body weight in a month. If I lost 5 percent (nine pounds) in a month, I'd be feeling pretty light and happy about it, but since weight is very easy to measure, we use it to measure our care.

Very old people seem like a separate species, but there are usually shards of dignity remaining underneath all the puckers and oddities. They may be stubborn, lazy, or impossible to decipher, but I'd say they have earned the right to do as they damn well please. I certainly don't think that I am in any position to truly know what they are experiencing within those gnarled and creaky bodies. I assume that like you and me, they normally feel urges to eat when they are hungry and to drink when they are thirsty. Basic human metabolism is largely self-regulating. Shutting down is a natural part of that self-regulating life cycle. Residents may also have a very legitimate urge to let go, to surrender to nature. And I don't know how it happened that we became the moral authorities over their biologies. These people have not changed their nature by becoming helpless. Their lives are miserable enough just from being confined here in Hotel Lonely. I look forward to the day when we will have enough courage and balance to trust human nature and to honor all its stages, including the end of it. Perhaps we feel uncomfortable with the prospect and vision of infirmity. Maybe we force the infirm to stay alive out of our own need to give succor. Perhaps our caregiving is more about us than them. At times dementia leads some to overeat and others not to eat at all. But how do we distinguish between dementia and the decline of digestion? I believe that sometimes life mercifully wants to end by means of its own choosing. Forcing a body to stay alive can be cruel.

When I first saw a 250-pound nurse stuffing food down an unwilling, protesting, pleading 70-pound resident I wanted to crawl under the table in embarrassment, but I dared not speak out. It was my second day on the job. That resident was Marlie. She repeatedly insisted that she didn't want anything to eat. After she was fed, she vomited her meal. The nurse said, "She makes herself do that."

Okay. But why?

More recently I watched in pain as Trudy (an aide) forced Luna, who is already quite obese, to eat food that she has rejected all her life. Luna just kept getting madder and madder. Trudy, I know, believes she was doing what's best for Luna. She was taught that the elderly must eat loads of calories to heal and maintain healthy skin. If they lose weight the facility is called on the carpet. Trudy has every excuse to force Luna to eat. Privately, I wonder how much nutrition Luna really absorbed with a bellyful of anger and humiliation.

There are other ways of looking at this. In India and China, traditional wisdom says that we must be calm and collected to eat and digest properly. Some claim that even the attitude of those preparing the food influences its nutritional value. Here when old people lose their appetite, we literally wash food down with bitter spirit, ignoring all the hormones we are producing when we "get their bile up." We can be so righteous, we wear our righteousness like a halo.

Recently the Dalai Lama was asked if he had any advice for America. He said, "Eat less." While he was still competing in body building, Arnold Schwarzenegger played in a movie based on a novel titled *Stay Hungry*. A little hunger is not a bad thing.

My point is that we are systematically not listening to these residents. By gorging those we care for like Sumo wrestlers, we violate their dignity just as we would by crudely withholding food. We focus on getting their bodies to act the way we want, even while their whole physical-mental-emotional system may be screaming at us to leave them alone and let them go gracefully in some other direction. We apply the rules as handed down regardless of the effect.

Oddly, we would rarely think of infringing on residents' rights by discouraging emphysema patients from smoking all they want, even though we all know it's self-destructive. Feeding residents can easily become a form of well-intentioned bullying.

One nurse said to me, "In effect we are their parents." I understand where that thought comes from. Typically old folks lose their abilities in reverse order to the way they gained them as infants and toddlers. "Geriatrics becomes pediatrics," to quote a local neurologist. Easing our way out of life often becomes a mirror image of how we come into it, and nursing homes do take care of these "children" as they lose control over their own bodies, function by function. However, my problem with that way of thinking is that along with parenthood comes the right to discipline: "Eat your vegetables or no TV for you!" Where does that right begin and end? How do we know what's best for them? And how good a job are we doing raising our fat young children anyway?

The first person I was assigned to feed was a woman in the back named Ruth. I met Ruth in the Surrey Dining Room, where we feed those residents who are more disturbing and less presentable. She was already advanced in some sort of dementia that caused her to squeeze her eyes tightly shut and to move and sway constantly from the hip, forward and back, and to thrust her arms and elbows in irregular yet rhythmic sweeps and jabs. So there I was, assigned to feed a moving target with her eyes squeezed shut. I noticed that every second or third lunge forward Ruth would open her mouth. So I timed my moves with a loaded spoon, and soon I learned that I could feed her this way. Then she began pushing her tongue forward to expel the oatmeal and liquefied toast I was giving her. (Yummy! Have another sip of toast, Ruth!) So I countered her tongue movement by keeping the spoon in her mouth a little longer. During all of this time I more or less assumed that I was dealing with a mind that was . . . well, more or less, less than more. Then Ruth abruptly opened her eyes, glared directly at me and said, "Goddammit!" Maybe she had privately discovered a secret dance previously held only by the whirling dervishes. Then along I come with spoonfuls of toast desecrating her kinetic rapture.

So what is gained by turning a miserable geriatric day into a terrible one? Only in nursing homes have I seen a systematic obesity program seen as evidence of good care. The conventional idea behind all this is that an abundance of nutrition is required to heal wounds (bedsores) and to maintain strength. Perhaps there is also something to be said for allowing one's digestion to take a rest occasionally. The body has to marshal tremendous resources to digest tough pork chops and wads of white bread and push them through a tired GI tract.

A centenarian once gave me this advice: "Leave the table a little bit hungry and you will have more energy in the ensuing hours. You will feel better. Try it."

Excuse this comparison. I have a dachshund that likes to chase cars. One day she finally caught one and came out of the encounter somewhat the worse for wear. After the initial shock, she curled up in a corner and could not be persuaded to eat anything for four days until her trauma was healed and she felt better. We trusted her to know what she needed most.

Similarly, zoo keepers typically feed mammals only two days out of three. Even small ruminants with their rapid metabolisms are said to live 30 percent longer with regularly imposed fasting. My point is that the body has a wisdom of its own; I suspect that we'd do well to trust our more primitive nature. Nature knows far more than our high-minded strategizing or ersatz maternal succor ever will.

Back to Reality

I, fed with judgement, in a fleshy tomb, am
Buried above ground.
—William Cowper (1731–1800)

Meanwhile, back at breakfast, Letha arrives in her chair wildly proclaiming, "The devil's loose! The devil's loose!" Dulcie sits alone at her isolated little table beside the wall, hunched over, constantly mumbling, "Hey, hey, hey," occasionally throwing her food on the floor when some phantasm privately displeases her. She hit Rebecca on the back of the head with a cup last week, so now we position her to face the wall. Bess politely approaches an unsuspecting visitor in the vestibule and tells him that a man was just shot out back and that we are selling thirteen-year-old girls in the shower room.

Mena, sitting with her flaming red hair swept back, appears to be coifed by a wind tunnel. Her delightfully sour face with its shark fin–like nose seems to be speeding even while she's sitting perfectly still. I greet her, "Hi, Mena." Mena squawks back suspiciously, "Well all right, but how high?" Three minutes later she recognizes me, "There he is, there's my black belt boy" (referring to the black back support all aides must wear). "I want some lemon milk! And I want it right now!" I ask her if she means coffee with cream in it. "Yes, and three of those little round things in it, too." "Okay, three creamers," I reply. Mena lays claim to all the clothing protectors. "They're all mine," she says, "every one of them. I bought them with my own money. You can use one if you want to, but I want them all back. I paid a lot of money for them, more than a dollar and a quarter each. You don't want to cheat people and then throw it right back at them . . ."

Calvin, who is blind and deaf, briefly stands up in the midst of the dining tables, unzips his fly, and relieves his bladder on the linoleum floor. A yellow Wet Floor cone is placed over the puddle. Later the kitchen staff will mop it up. Gilda looks intently down at her plate and tells me that she is afraid of her potatoes. Doreen rocks in her wheelchair, eyes shut tight in a private rapture, caresses her lap, and moans, "Awwwm, I need eighteen inches. Awww . . ." Luna feeds herself fairly well, though half the time she misses her mouth by half an inch to the left. Mariah stabs her cereal with a spoon as if she's trying to kill it, but then shuts her mouth tightly when a food-laden spoon is offered to her. Then she wraps her egg sandwich neatly in a paper napkin and turns to the woman seated next to her and offers it as a gift with an ad-lib aria, "I lo-o-ve you, I lo-o-ve yooou." Melka reaches into her sweatpants but is blocked by the wheelchair armrests. "I itch . . . I itch . . . I itch," she says. "Please, somebody scratch my ass." Meanwhile dainty little Paulette is content to quietly water the plastic flowers in the brick planter by the window.

Marcus, who is ninety-six and never took a piano lesson in his life sits down at the piano and begins to play. He calms us all with an endless series of melodies that effortlessly flow out of his hands without a forethought. If you ask him about it, he denies that he knows anything about music. But the music from his hands, anything from "Let Me Call You Sweetheart" to Monto-

vani, calms and soothes us and somehow seems to pull the sur-
real dining hall scene together.

I stand up straight and survey the room. I crane my neck like
a prairie dog on lookout duty. I see that eventually we shall live
inside a Fellini film.

Before most of the residents have even been served breakfast,
Marge flags me down, waving her stiff, withered hand and ur-
gently demanding, "Tom, I really have to go the bathroom."
When Marge calls me, she has a way of sounding quite urgent
and demanding, beckoning me as if we were tree-house playmates but, at the same time, instructing me I'd better get my butt
over there right quick if I know what's good for me. I feel as
though I know what it was like to be her child, to grow up under her wrathful affection. When I move in close, she talks to me
as if she's sharing a secret. I wheel her down the long hall as she
grumbles, "I wouldn't feed my dog the crap they give us here. It's
enough to gag a maggot on a gut wagon!" She may even pro-
claim, "I am never going to eat in that dining hall again. Never!"
I nod, suggesting agreement with her, but actually, I find the food
surprisingly tasty here.

"When we get down to my room we'll pig out. If you don't
take something to eat, I'm going to have to beat you . . . again."
Marge sees her sweet favors as her single means to bring our
friendship to a satisfying balance. It's her hook. If I forget to pick
up my Dolly Madison fruit pie, Marge continues to call me to
her side to remind me. She badgers me with her offering until I
accept.

We roll into her room, I reach over her shoulder to open the
bathroom door ahead of us then swing my foot behind to kick
the outer door closed. Entry door, bathroom door, and closet
door in every room clash against each other in an architectural

feud of door clanging, gouged wood veneers, and scarred varnish. The owners built five nursing homes previous to this one. I joke to Marge that they needed a lot of practice to get the architecture this wrong.

I lock her chair wheels in front of the toilet, lift her by her armpits, pivot her on her wooden leg (which is much stronger than her real leg), pull down her slacks and panties as she grips me in a half nelson and ease her down onto the pot. I try not to pull on her pubic hair as my hand passes by the privacy zone to remove the panty liner. I slump for a minute into her wheelchair, waiting as she pees. "It's kind of hard to piss in front of a nice looking young man," she says. We smile at each other in a knowing camaraderie and mutual acceptance of our absurd relationship. She bellows out a flabby, wet fart that echoes roundly from the toilet bowl. I make some joke about her stepping on a frog or my fanciful threat of placing a microphone inside the toilet bowl for the world to hear her bluster. Giving me a tired smile she says, "Well, I guess I'm done." I step up and don a rubber glove. I grab hold of her armpits and hoist her up from behind to a nearly erect position, bracing both of her arms onto the wheelchair armrests. I position both my legs around hers. For balance I clinch her with my knees as she leans forward; I wipe her butt, flush down the dirty toilet paper, pull up her panties and fresh pantyliner and then her slacks. She tells me, "Pull those up over my gut will you, hon?" Then from behind I cradle my forearms under her armpits and pivot her around, pull the empty wheelchair in as close as I can with one foot, and plop her down in her seat with a heavy thud. "You're going to hurt yourself some day doing that, dammit. Then I'll have to whip you again."

"I don't guess they brought me any ice water yet, have they?" she asks. "Not yet," I respond. We have the same exchange every day. "Take me in there and get me something to eat from the middle drawer, will you, hon? I'm hungry as a bitch wolf in heat." She freely lets all the world know how much she suffers to be here, swallowing the indignity of dependence. I roll her over to her standard-issue three-drawer dresser of particle board and plastic photo-wood-grain veneer, reach down, and fish out a Reese's peanut butter cup. The drawer falls out of its failed polyvinyl T-guide rail every time. I peel the candy wrapper and give it to her. Then I struggle to realign the drawer out of its fractured position. Marge's sisters regularly import a supply of sugary snacks for her. All four of her sisters come to see her, wearing their stern, scowling faces and unkempt country hair. The whole family sports an in-your-face demeanor, but after several months we've warmed up to each other. Nonetheless, I agree with the front-office wisdom that this whole clan is best not to be trifled with. I make small talk and consent to whatever the family says.

Marge is a serious diabetic but we allow her the freedom to poison herself all she likes. She's fully aware of her choices. "Most diabetics are crazy for sweets," she says confidently, her mouth overstuffed with peanut butter cups, "but not me."

"Take me out of this place or just shoot me here, I don't care which," she comments as she chomps down the Reese's in two ravaging bites. "Many times I've wanted to roll my wheelchair outside and over that cliff," she says.

"That little drop-off out back is no more than three feet deep," I retort. Marge looks down, screws her face into a feigned snarl, and grumbles in disappointment. Another escape fantasy foiled by cruel reality.

I give her a swig of water to wash the sugar down, wheel her back up to the top of the hall, park her on Marty's left. Sometimes they offer each other a stick of chewing gum. If Marge sees that Marty is already chewing one of her own, she might ask in the falsetto manner of a hillbilly child, "Can I chew your gum for awhile?" Then they resume their stakeout duties. Within minutes they are both sound asleep.

One day I took Marge out for a long drive. We toured her old neighborhood down by the river ten or twelve miles north of here. She showed me the house she'd lived in. "They still got those ugly curtains I put up thirty years ago." We ran into an old neighbor who lived behind her all that while, but the old lady's lights had dimmed and she didn't recognize Marge. She showed me where she used to go skinny-dipping in the river as a brazen school kid. I was looking forward to treating Marge to any kind of food her tortured heart desired. I wanted to relieve this harried woman's constant complaints about the quality of food at the nursing home. "Anything at all, I'm game to treat you. Wherever you want to go." Marge responded glumly, "I'm not hungry," refusing to become indebted.

So we just drove around for a couple of hours. After a time she said that her mother used to cook new potatoes with peas and how much she loved them. Of course I had no access to her mother's new potatoes and peas, so Marge remained safe, holding on to her sense of deprivation. After all, if I took her deprivation away she would have nothing left to protect herself from openly accepting her dependence on strangers and her loss of power. As we neared "the home" on our return, I told her that I'd rather she didn't tell Marty that we went out, because I could not do the same for her, her body being all twisted and frozen as it is. She no longer fits in cars. I didn't want her to be jealous or disappointed. Marge objected, "You're taking all the fun out of this for me," but she seemed to agree. On the way back Marge thanked me seven times (I counted) for taking her out.

The first thing Marty said to me, after I'd sneaked Marge back in front of her TV to catch the end of her soaps, was "I heard you and Marge eloped."

Months later I heard that an aide had taken it upon herself to quiz Marge about our outing, suspecting that I took her out for purposes of sexual molestation. Marge ran that aide out of the room.

Marty's physical therapist is from India, a woman named Kindu. At lunch one day Marty rhymed,

> Kindu, the Hindu
> If by chance, she loses her pants,
> She'll have to let her skin do.

I shared this with Kindu. Marty was upset with me for sharing her private slander.

Marty often wears shorts. Her metabolism runs high, she sweats profusely, and she's usually warm to the touch. She also likes a chance to show off her legs. She is still proud of her fine complexion; it is her one proud possession. A few other residents raise objections to this immodest display of flesh, but nobody pays them much heed. Occasionally a truly demented lady like Audrey or Thelma will approach Marty and begin to affectionately stroke her legs or give her unintelligible compliments and observations. This gives Marge an opportunity to defend Marty, and she relishes the role. Marge will spew out her vitriol on the intruder, who most often remains totally unaware of being scolded. Neither Marty nor Marge can actually do anything physical to halt the invasion of their space. The fingers on Marge's right hand are permanently curled inward by diabetic neuropathy to form a weak fist, so when she gets really angry she'll wave her fist and hump up and down on her haunches while shaking with frustration. If she sees me on the hall she'll start yelling, "Tom! Tom! Get her the hell out of here!" Likely as not, the offending intruder is led away or simply pointed in another direction, still unaware of even being addressed.

Alzheimer's victims, dubbed "All-timers" by fellow residents, may wake up to a new world every time they blink. This makes them exceptionally forgiving human beings. I often find their presence refreshing and pleasant.

Marty tells me that she and Marge knew each other casually all through their early married years. Their husbands both worked for the same power company for decades. Marty admits that Marge takes good care of her, but she is offended by her language.

"If she ever cussed me like that I'd slap the shit out of her and then I'd slap her for shitting," boasts Marty.

Marge privately tells me that Marty is "going downhill fast. She cries like a baby at the silliest damn thing." Occasionally Marge will have me take her to her room just to get away from Marty's incessant "Does my son still live at Indian Lake? What time is it?"

She criticizes Marty's emotional dependence on her son, Bert. To Marge's mind, Bert's two-week trip out West mutates into "a four month vacation without her. If any kin of mine took off on a trip for four months, he'd a known better than to come back— *ever!* That silly Marty was so happy just to see him when he got back, I couldn't stand to watch it. She was happy just to see the pictures he took!"

Occasionally Marty will call me over to her Geri-Chair to say, "I shit my britches," or "I need my pants changed." This is not fun for us or for Marty. She feels embarrassed. Changing her is usually a two- or even three-person job. Her knees are held stiffly together, and when loads of brown stuff are squished up into her privates—well, it gets pretty clinical. Marty deals with this assault on her pride by zoning out. She gets that glazed look in her eyes as we roll her stiff body back and forth on her bed, prying her knees apart. Her expression seems to say, "I don't understand what's happening to me. Is this real?"

It seems to those of us who work with her that Marty has long ago given up on herself. For years she has felt that she was doomed. From the onset she has refused to take the recommended steps to help herself in even the slightest way, even to slow the progress of her contracting muscles and her contracting world. She would have nothing to do with therapy. In fact, her son once said that the moment Marty heard her diagnosis, sixteen years ago, she just caved in and has not done anything to help herself since. It was the diagnosis that made her stop moving, long before the disease itself froze her muscles and joints. The implosion of her will locked her on a downward spiral, an ever accelerating eddy of decline.

Perhaps I would react the same way if I believed that God Himself had condemned me. Marty told me that not long after she became a marked woman, a friendly nurse advised her to exercise her hands or they would turn into claws. Marty admits that she refused to believe the nurse. But now her hands are claws. They cannot be pried open by any humane means. Marty steadfastly refuses physical therapy treatments to open her hands up even to insert a small swatch of cloth. Therapy is not asking for much of a stretch, just enough to keep her fingernails from slowly digging holes in her palms from the constant pressure. She proclaims her refusal by wailing, and invariably we consent to her emotional tyranny rather then disrupt an entire wing of the building. She refuses to allow us to put her in a more upright position in her Geri-Chair (to permit her to look forward and not have to stare at the ceiling all day long). She's more comfortable soaking in the bath of her own misery while avoiding the eyes of casual passers-by. Misery has become her home, her lover, and her warm and nurturing mother.

It appears that a part of her wants to be coddled and pitied and doted over. In her theology, her regrettable condition requires us to pity her and thus do whatever she wants. Her demands are stated matter-of-factly and, to be fair, they are not at all offensive in tone. Nonetheless, I cannot recall that I have ever heard her say please or thank you to anyone. I mentioned this observation to her once. She said, "You don't have to say please in a place like this." As a result, her fits of crying, which can come up from being abandoned for all of two or three minutes, irritate staff and residents alike, but she keeps it up because it gets her what she wants. Her crying is so loud that we cannot tolerate it for long without responding. One nurse staged a resistance to her pathos for a time. Marty told me, "I hate her guts." In short order Marty won out.

Marty is a good Baptist. She firmly believes that Parkinson's disease is God's punishment of her. She doesn't know why, but He surely must hold a heinous grudge against her to clinch her in the grips of such a terrible disease. Perhaps in her world it has become her duty and her right to suffer bitterly. She feels herself going down an irreversible spiral. Parkinson's disease *is* merciless. It seems to take its victims on a headlong and fully conscious path into a premature rigor mortis, an active mind trapped inside a frozen body. Arms and legs steadfastly refuse to take orders. Marty watched as her hands became as fixed as bale hooks, the progress irreversible. As her body becomes more and more rigid, her emotions become more and more labile, her future more and more bleak.

She is seeing her malignancy solidify daily. Her muscles ache. She said to me once, "This is not science fiction." She wonders aloud, "Why is this happening to me?"

I went to Wal-Mart and bought a Walkman with Marty in mind. Then I brought in some meditative relaxation tapes for her. I hoped to influence her mind-set, but she was not interested.

Marty is chained in hell—real, concrete horror beyond the pale of anything Edgar Allan Poe could concoct when he imagined what it was like to be buried alive. Parkinson's is being calcified alive; Marty is becoming the proverbial pillar of salt.

When Marty's visitors arrive—extended family or neighbors from times past—she breaks out in pitiful fits of tears. Her howls tend to cut short the mood of any intended festivities. I can say something as innocuous as "Bert is a really good man," and Marty will immediately break down.

In quiet and unexpected moments I might slap her thigh smartly or even give her a quick peck on the cheek for no reason at all. She might smile warmly, or she might look at me as though I am from Mars. Nonetheless, when I get fed up with working here and threaten to quit, Marty says, "If you quit, I'm moving to another nursing home." That kind of talk is flattering for a moment, but I doubt that it means much. We all know this momentary affection cannot translate into action, because like most residents she is in command of nothing but her own disposition. I take her threat to transfer as a belated thank-you.

The dining hall needs to be cleared of residents as quickly as possible so it can be bused, washed down, and vacuumed. There is a constant stream of wheelchairs going out and late arrivals coming in. Nurses count and crush pills and aides help residents eat—lifting laden forks, cutting up meat, pouring coffee, wiping chins, dabbing up spilled milk. Residents raise their hands and beg to be exited or just yell for help to be taken off their sore butts, wheeled to their rooms, and laid down. For most residents, sleep is the sweetest commodity we can provide.

Unfortunately, in most cases we cannot permit unlimited sleep. If residents are allowed to sleep for as long as they want in their habitual positions, they become weak, their skin breaks down in spots where circulation is cut off by the constant pressure, or they can catch pneumonia. When residents die we're forced to close our account with that family. No more money. And, as always, we are under the watchful eye of the state. I have seen no instance where we willingly hasten the death of anyone. Yet we seem incapable of dealing with the fact that some people are on friendly terms with death. This says more about our fears than about the residents'.

Nonetheless, I do go out of my way to lay Millicent down because she is in such pain. She is not a resident in my hall, but she has the face of an angel. Her smile is truly beatific, and her considerable wits are all about her. She has a master's degree in business and made a good deal of money in her life. She owns four hundred acres inside the city limits. Her son ran for the Senate, but he came in a distant second in the primaries. A few years ago, when she lost her health, she was left lying in her bed far too long and got a terrible bedsore on her coccyx. Most of the flesh atrophied and was eaten away down there, which means that today she sits on scar tissue and bone. It takes me only a few extra minutes to wheel Millicent down and plop her in bed, stuff a pillow under one side to relieve pressure on her coccyx, and spread some Bag Balm on her scars to relieve the pain. As I lean over to transfer her she says, "Oh, thank heavens." As I lift her up she playfully recites, "Stand . . . twist . . . squat." She is so grateful. "My butt thanks you," and then once: "I don't know why you take such good care of me." I have no reply for her because she's an avowed atheist, or so she claims, and has no supporting beliefs. I cannot give her a good reason. I give her my best smile. "Try to behave for ten minutes," I tease and then I go.

I overheard Millie and a nurse talk about another resident who'd been failing. The nurse informed her that the other resident had died the previous night, "But we shouldn't feel sad because the Bible says we should rejoice when a soul goes to our true home in heaven."

Millie said, "Ah, don't bother me with the Bible. The Bible is full of shit." The good nurse went pale and nearly buckled in shock. Unable to regain her composure, she found no words to respond. But one morning on the way to her bed, Millie kept repeating, "Oh thank you, God. Oh thank you, God."

I said to her, "I thought you were an atheist."

"Not this morning," she replied.

One day she complained about an itch in her pubic area. She laughed, "I think I got crabs. My grandpa came home with crabs every time he went to the whorehouse to get his bean snapped."

On a later morning Millie was visibly worried and said to me, "I hope they make sure I'm dead when they cremate me. I sure would hate to wake up in all those flames." I assured her that it's easy to tell when someone is truly dead and that she didn't have much to worry about.

At one point Millie became quite ill with an infection. Anxiety and confusion followed. In a state of terror she insisted over and over, "I'm dead. I'm dead."

I got in close and told her, "Millie, you're delusional."

She said, "Oh."

The next day she laughed and thanked me. That first time this approach worked with her. But subsequent attempts, when the delusion reappeared, failed.

Millicent's roommate is Doreen, and she's a hoot. She had a major stroke. One hand is drawn up tight and close-fisted against her chest, and one eye always seems closed. She often seems lucid. The one thing that distinguishes her is a profound and unabashed habit of masturbating quite openly in any location and without a hint of embarrassment. Doreen also entertains us with her mysterious vocalizations. She will speak quite clearly at times, repeating phrases such as, "O Medusa, come to me, Medusa," or she might just as easily repeat, "Potato, O Potato," in such a seductive tone as to suggest that she has a secret romance with tubers.

I wheel Bud and Walter back to their room and turn on Bud's thirteen-inch black-and-white TV. I lock their chairs and clamp a call button cord within their reach. Then I struggle to give them a quick shave. Shaving the men is a favorite elective activity for me. Maybe it's a guy thing. Doing battle with wild men, I wield a sharp blade against the folds of a gruff cheek. I smooth it over and calm it down. But I might not enjoy it as much if they were compliant. I am delighted by residents who have fight left in them. Bud tries to stall, "Well, now . . . wait a minute. Goddamn it! Where's Walter?"

"Can I shave you, Bud? Maybe your daughter is coming today. You want to look good, don't you?"

"Well, yeah . . . but only on Tuesss . . . day."

He lets me shave him if I go slowly enough, until I come to a sensitive area around his lips. Then he violently throws his head left and right, cussing all the way. I let him cuss and grouse and I keep on scraping. His fussing is over in a few minutes.

I make their beds. Most often these boys are quite free with their urine, but not always. Some days go more smoothly than others for no apparent reason, other than a full moon or a plague of diarrhea.

After his shave Walter pulls himself along the wooden handrails that line the halls, slowly proceeding in his chair until he reaches a spot of sunlight at the far end where sheets of plate glass replace concrete blocks. He gratefully bows his head and falls immediately to sleep. If I am lucky the urine slowly dribbling inside his diaper will not leak out until after lunch.

Bud will sit in his chair watching television without the slightest clue what is on, or he will just sit. It seems to make no difference. We have no idea if *I Love Lucy* reaches all the way into his brain or not. He could be in a yogic trance. If I ask him a question, he has a way of sounding relaxed and at ease with the situation. He might ask, "Where's Walton?" or "Where's Wilber?" even while looking directly at Walter just three feet away. Walter, of course, has no idea who Bud is. Nonetheless Bud gives the impression of being really attached to his roommate and concerned about his welfare. I ask Bud how he's doing. "Pure D," he says, "Pure D, easy money." I have no idea what he means by this. Bud appears content—as long as we leave him alone, that is. He waves me aside and says he wants to introduce me to his good friend, but he can't remember the man's name. Then Bud sits and watches the day go by.

I like to put Libby on the pot whenever I get the chance. We steal a quiet moment of friendship. It seems as if we've known each other forever. She is among the most even-tempered women I've met.

Her wardrobe is oddly limited by color. Almost all her clothes are fire-engine red. Libby was a real "Rosie the Riveter" during the Second World War. She built bomber parts in Los Angeles. When she was growing up during the Depression her entire family had to eat possum. "What did that taste like?" I asked. "Well," she smiles coolly, "I haven't eaten it since." Two of her children died young, one in a fire and the other in a river, or so she says. Libby has a little palsy in her right arm; her hand shakes constantly. If I give her hand something to hold, the shaking usually stops. Despite many tragedies in her life, she somehow chooses to patiently bide her time, seeming to accept a fate that would defeat a lesser woman. Libby enjoys herself; she seems not to have an ounce of resistance or resentment in her. I make a point of hugging her and giving her a kiss. Conversing with her has the feel of rocking chairs and long-eared dogs lounging on the back stoop, and the relaxed, down-home quality of her voice comforts me.

But then, a while back, Libby pulled me aside and asked confidentially, "How come you didn't come by last night? I stayed up till past eleven." A day or two later she began to worry about "the baby beside me in bed." My mind begins to question if we have any kind of real relationship at all. I go out into the hall puzzled and somewhat saddened.

Occasionally I give Adrian a ride to his room. He announces in his stentorian voice, "I've got to pisszz." He drags out the s for a dramatic, in-your-face emphasis. And while on the pot, if he's having a little bowel trouble he pronounces, "Bring me that fat nurse, that really fat one."

Adrian comes off as arrogant and demanding. He gave me a hard time until I acted angry with him one time and insisted that he consider the twenty-five other residents I also have to care for. After that I became one of his favorites, and since then he has pretty much left me in peace. He also appreciated the fact that my Case brand pocketknife held a keen edge when he asked to borrow it one morning to open mail from his stockbroker. He smiled at it with an approving nod as he felt the blade.

During virtually every breakfast Midge leaves early to have a BM explosion in her pants and needs to be cleaned up. If I'm lucky I beat her colon's clock and get her on the pot before she lies down and defiles her bedclothes. Ro needs to be pottied before she lies down; Barb needs to be turned; Harold gets fed in his room. Marge screams for my attention, "Tom, . . . come here." She waves me in closer, then whispers, "You know, I haven't been to the bathroom since eight o'clock last night." It's a busy time.

Meanwhile breakfast is still progressing. Stella sucks up her pureed mush through a straw. Liquefied eggs, biscuits, and the whatever du jour can be spooned into her milk, swirled into a uniform gray-brown consistency, and then administered through a straw. It's about the only way she'll eat.

Pop comes late to breakfast. Pop is an utterly unique case. He has been retired from government work for forty-seven years. He's over a hundred years old, and he lives on a back hall with his ninety-six-year-old wife, Eliza, who seems to be always roaming the halls looking for him. The two of them make a great couple. "Oh, I'm so happy you're with me, baby," he says after she finds him, most likely taking a nap in some stranger's bed. And I am certain he means it. He wears a tattered cowboy hat or a baseball cap emblazoned with the phrase "The older I get, the better I was."

When a pretty blonde aide helps get him up in the morning, Pop closes his eyes and takes hold of her waist with both hands and thrusts his hips forward and back saying, "Ooo, baby! Come on, baby, I really want to go to bed with you." But when Pop once spied me casually putting a hand on his wife's shoulder, he got jealous. He started telling the women that I'm no good. After eating breakfast he sits in his wheelchair and flutters his feet at a rapid pace to propel himself forward down the hall looking for the nearest available bed, or he might stand up as best he can behind his wife's chair. He gives her a push down the long hall.

Or if he lets me push him back to his room he talks constantly with great joy and enthusiasm, "Oh, man, we're really going now. Oh yeah, man, you really know how to do it. Haaa ha!" Pop chews on the flat end of an unlit foot-long cigar. He tells his wife again, "I sure am glad you're with me, I sure am glad. Ha haaa!"

Not long ago I saw him throw his food on the dining room floor. I quickly wheeled him back to his room to lay him down, and I asked him if he was mad when he did that. "No," he said, "I was just having fun."

It was also during breakfast that I found Enoch dead in his bed on 500 Hall. His roommate, Casper, had asked for help, so I wheeled him to his bed. And there was Enoch, still as an ocher statue. I had intended to check on Enoch since I'd heard his health was declining. His wife had stayed up all night with him and then she went home for only half an hour to shower and change clothes. Enoch must have died just a few minutes before she returned. He was still warm when I found him. His body didn't look so bad, really. He just wasn't breathing. When his wife got to his bedside, she cradled his head in her arms, kissed him, and said, "Oh, sweetheart, I'm going to miss you so."

Flora had become a familiar fixture at the nursing home. A loyal wife, for more than a year she came every day to visit Enoch and spent almost all day there. She was a convivial person to have around.

Enoch served as a photographer in the Second World War. He flew twenty-some missions over Tokyo, photographing the aftermath of our fire bombing. Afterward he became an electrical engineer. He contracted Parkinson's shortly after retirement, and it gradually, quietly froze the life out of him.

Enoch was too far advanced when I started working here for

me to get to know him. I never heard him speak, never saw him walk. They say that little more than a year ago he was walking up and down the halls, talkative, vital, astute, and humorous.

But now here he was, his body cooling down, a single tear pooled in one eye socket. Another aide and I rolled a towel and propped it under his chin to help hold his mouth shut. We tried to straighten his legs out, but they had been contracted far too long to give up their hold. Another aide said they'd have to cut his tendons to get him into a casket (not so, according to the local mortician).

Back out in the hall, Flora reflected for a moment on their satisfying marriage. She recalled that when she turned forty he told her that he was going to trade her in for two twenties. Pleased with herself, she told him, "You're not wired for two-twenty."

After Breakfast

After breakfast we aides check out our daily assignment sheets and coordinate how we will divide our chores—giving baths, taking weights, getting vitals (pulse, blood pressure), turning Barb, moving Harold from bed to chair and back, shaving, grooming, and above all, pottying.

When I work with Reba I'm 50 percent sure we will have a good day. Reba is not afraid to work. So many aides are lackluster, but not this one. She goes full steam ahead. Reba would boss God right to his face if she could get her arms around him. Twenty-three years old, five-feet-four, and 197 pounds of muscle and sinew, she is undauntable. I envy her shoulders. Her biceps are solid as bricks. I love her direct manner.

Zelda hates it. When Zelda wanted Reba to treat her vaginal irritation, Reba objected flatly: "I'm not going to put Vaseline on your pussy." She loves to put Zelda in her place, which means anything but the special treatment most staff tend to give her so reluctantly. Reba got straight A's in a tiny backwoods school in Appalachia. Surprisingly, she also learned to love opera there. Presently she lives in a rundown trailer with her new husband and drives six hours every other weekend to fight for custody of her little boy. As coworkers, our personalities complement each other. Whereas I like to placate and to please, Reba lays it out straight, orders everyone around, and relishes irritating those who displease her.

Her greetings are informal. She slugs me on the shoulder or socks me in the gut, sending me a fist out of nowhere, knocking the wind out of me, and by this I know she's having a good day. At the same time she can be tender and caring toward the helpless, and on some lucky residents she lavishes love and tenderness. She quietly buys them underwear, makeup, and doodads for their hair. This she does while taking home an even lower wage that I do. In her case a quarter of it goes to child support and thousands of dollars to lawyer fees.

Reba's present husband, Gene, comes in often, bringing a sack lunch, sometimes flowers. He is tall, narrow shouldered, and hyper-energetic. Vietnam gave him a few extra facial crags and tics. He is exceptionally long in the tooth. Every month or so he shows up minus another incisor or canine. Finally he came in with a new set of dentures. You could see he felt dressed up, but these bargain models were so oversized that he could barely pull his lips over them. They gave him a horselike appearance, but of course I didn't say anything. Gene's disposition is surprisingly upbeat, and he's full of country humor. He holds his thumb and forefinger about an inch apart and says, "If I squeezed the shit out of that woman, there wouldn't be but that much left to her." She stares at him smiling broadly, "Just try it, buster."

Reba's affections are erratic and uneven, however. She will endear herself to one of us and then without explanation emotionally abandon the unsuspecting soul, who is left to wonder what went wrong.

Tinker went through Reba's hot-cold cycle twice before she talked to me about it. True to her self-flagellating fashion, Tinker asked me, "Do you think Reba is jealous about me and you?"

Reba and I exchange friendly insults. She beats on me. When

she disappears or just stops hitting me, I know something must be wrong. I wait for the return of her good graces when she smacks me hard, unawares, knocking the living wind out of me from around a blind corner, and struts off laughing. I wipe Mariah's butt cheek with a washcloth, then lob it toward Reba's face. She lops a glob of A&D ointment on my hair. I spritz the bottom of her shorts, to make it look like she wet herself. But when I offer to make a character statement in her favor for the judge in Nashville, I notice that Reba's eyes water in tacit appreciation.

I know when she is dealing with trouble because she pulls away, escaping emotionally. Reba can be social and happy one minute and pushy and spiteful the next. I find her tack impossible to decipher and, in time, I lose interest in trying to win back her playful onslaughts.

Oddly, I discover that this makes no difference to her whatsoever. She is happy one minute, angry the next regardless of what I may do. I begin to understand that the puzzlement of working with her is my problem and has no impact on her at all. Reba is Reba. You take her or leave her. She doesn't care much one way or the other, or so she would have us believe.

Right before and right after meals is "potty time." It is the time to prevent accidents. We have seventeen people who, we are told, must be pottied every two hours. That strict requirement has never been met. That's not possible at this staffing level.

A locally prominent social worker told me that incontinence is the most common reason old folks are put in nursing homes. Others maintain the most common single reason for admission to long-term care is a broken hip.

It takes a lot to keep up with leaky valves. I lift and strip lots of heavy butts. I put them on the pot and let them sit and dribble for awhile. A few residents will potty themselves. Some get off the potty on their own but have to be coaxed to get on. Others who can do nothing for themselves will ask to go potty just to relieve the boredom.

Betty would live in the bathroom if we let her. Right after breakfast she makes her way there and begins stripping her clothes off, dealing with phantom grunts (BMs) and her irritation with her chair alarm. She cannot be convinced that any of her clothes are clean and dry. She frequently asks for a stick to help work out an imagined impaction. Or maybe she is impacted in her upper colon, out of our reach. Other residents cannot go while sitting or lying down but leak as soon as they are stood upright. A lot of wet shoes are the result. Marge always develops an urgent need to be pottied when her sisters arrive for a visit. She's usually extra ornery about it, too, more demanding than usual. I do not know if she is showing her sisters that she has a slave to do her dirty work or if she just needs to get away from the presence of her family for a few minutes.

Aides do not gain points for doing these tasks; we only lose points for not doing them. We have a schedule to maintain—prescribed routines to follow and tasks to perform and record. All the other stuff, what I would consider our real purpose, is officially just by-product.

All the affection, all the consoling, all the filling of emotional holes and the tidying up of frayed feelings are invisible to the owners, to the administration, and to the official state regulators who monitor us so closely. The heart is impossible to legislate, measure, or chart, but that, as we discover, doesn't make it any less vital or real. I have never known of any aide being rewarded or recognized for being kind. Yet I see it around me all the time. In general I will trust the heart of an aide over any other kind of worker. I know this is a very broad statement, but: so many aides are selfless givers, which means they are easily used.

Aching Hearts

Fortunately the bulk of our work is done behind closed doors, beyond the need for explanations, beyond the realm of measurements and records. What happens behind some doors is a lavish amount of blunt and raw comforting. I lay my head on residents' shoulders. I touch my forehead against theirs while I stare straight into their eyes at point-blank range. These acts trespass the conventional zone of private space. I do anything I can to give them just a few seconds of personal recognition. Doing this makes us both real for the moment. I meet these odd-looking folk as a coequal fellow adult, as a kissin' cousin or as their raucous adolescent, or godchild or executor . . . in whatever way they imagine me. I get as personal and close with these folks as I can. I believe that recognizing these residents individually, one at a time, is as welcome to them as rain in the desert. This is my technique, my joy, and my infirmity, a natural effusion of my own peculiar character mixed with an extraordinarily compelling environment. Only here in this place of ultimate desolation do I find the freedom to be so unguarded, so playful with so many people. Working in a nursing home brought this out of me. I was not a particularly open person before I started working here.

I am proud to be free within these confines. Other

aides may have other ways with other benefits. The way I do my job is very high maintenance. It slows me down. I spoil the lot of them. Here in this gritty place, reeling from fumes, in America's Point Zero, I have become a grownup child. I have learned what is really important to me, here on my knees in the dirt, afraid to be seen.

The great pain, the gut-wrenching void of nursing-home life has little to do with old age or infection or dementia. The dominant reality in our nursing home is ubiquitous separation. Mother Teresa once commented that the most serious epidemic in America is loneliness.

Everyone here is torn away from home and families. Publicly we call this "their home." This is in fact where residents lay their heads night after night, but a nursing home is rarely where the heart resides. How many real homes are attended by uniformed gatekeepers, as this one is? How many homes operate with the same bulk-rate, sterilized, cost-effective assembly-line efficiency we do?

I try to alleviate that institutional reality by directly attending to rampant loneliness. "My" residents are easily won over. There is nothing special about the way I give my service other than my repeated indulgence of being present to people. In my search for compassion I have concluded that "personal space" is a hellish prison. We adults sentence ourselves to social conventions.

Face to face, up close and personal, I learn to focus my full attention in flashes. One moment at a time, out comes my inner child. When I happen to touch residents softly or treat them affectionately, something may melt within and they become temporarily free of these depressing walls. We make contact. Our eyes lock as if to say, "Hi, I'm in here. What's it like in there where you are?" Their countenance relaxes. They love me. At various moments, I become someone they can relate to. Lucid or not, I am with them, a younger version of them, no better and no worse, barely different at all.

We all start out the same and we end up the same. All the differences that seem so important in life—the status, the achievements—are eventually reduced on our headstones to the hyphen inscribed between the year of our birth and the year of our death.

"All-timers," especially, live from moment to moment. I give them a moment of my heart and they take me in as one of their own. I become their social property. I love their free-wheeling world. I enter not so much as a particular individual but as an affectionate tone of voice or a familial echo or a zone of comfort. I also know just how easy it is to treat a helpless body like a sack of potatoes when time is rushed. I've done that too.

I can barely imagine the isolation and confusion I would feel as one of my own residents. What if some indifferent stranger in a white uniform suddenly flipped on the light and woke me up in the middle of a sweet dream. Not knowing where I am, not knowing what time of the day it is or what season is advancing outside, I would be totally confused. Defenseless, I would watch the stranger hurriedly pull sweatpants over my aching and stiff legs while I lie flat on my back. I might not recognize the clothes covering my arms and legs. Colors are dull, vision blurry, sounds muffled. I would see pictures on the walls. They might seem familiar and comfort me somewhat, but they might also seem off-key, strange. I'd know that this place is not exactly my home, but where am I?

Everything around me happens too fast. I wonder where my kids are or why Mom isn't here to hold me. Half-formed thoughts do not make it all the way to my mouth. I can't find the right words; I hear myself mumble. Who put me here? What's going on? Questions about my family are met with an indifferent shrug at best. Then the room spins and I find myself whirling through the air and suddenly sitting in a wheelchair in a hallway in a huge building where endless walls all look the same. Is this a prison? Am I sick? Are they doing experiments on me? Did I commit a crime? I nod off for a second and again I am someplace I've never seen before—or have I?

Later I watch another stranger absentmindedly raise a spoonful of something brown to my mouth. I swallow it obligingly. No taste. Maybe it's food, maybe it's poison. It just appears before me. I cannot tell what it is. After a few spoonfuls I want to stop. I have no appetite for any of this, but the young woman insists, so I go along, not knowing what she'll do to me if I resist. Thick liquid slides down my chin, my neck, and my undershirt, where it dries. My pants are wet. I cannot find my wallet. How will I pay for this? I am used to paying my own way.

I cannot find my keys. Where's the car? Nothing looks familiar. I see these strangers talking to each other while ignoring my questions. These strangers in white act like I'm some kind of ghost. Am I dead? I can't get through to them. I can tell they are unhappy about something, and I wonder what I did to be put here. Finally one of the white coats responds to me, puts a hand on my shoulder, and talks to me as though I were a small child. If I become too insistent and stir up a fuss, they give me a little pill. Everything gets heavy. I still do not know anything. Soon I couldn't care less. I slump forward in my wheelchair, unable to lift myself upright. My mouth goes dry, I feel dreamy, and I can't quite stay awake.

Everyone in white, all the people in control seem to buzz about very quickly. Wheelchairs speed down the hall at a reckless pace. Meanwhile, everything I do for myself has to be slow and careful, lest an accident occur. If I happen to find an exit door, an alarm goes off and the white coats turn me around. If I try to stand up, I am sternly ordered, "Sit down!" by someone no older than my grandkids. Some of these strangers begin to look familiar, but every few hours they are replaced by a completely different set of strangers.

Finally, they put me to bed. I feel clothes being peeled off. I'm cold, constantly cold. As I am lifted up, my foot scrapes against the chair pedal and I yell. My ribs hurt from the crush of dropping onto the bed. My protests make them mad at me. Bed at last. The weight of even holding up my head is off me. Thank God. Maybe I'll wake up and be home again.

In the dead of night the lights come on and a stranger in white puts a cold hand where I would never allow anyone, not even my mate, to touch me. Then I'm told I have messed the bed. I am mortified as they roll my naked body first left then right, spray me with something cold, and then wipe me off and strip my bed. Then just as suddenly they snap off their rubber gloves and disappear.

All that I have worked for and all those I have cherished for years have disappeared. I wonder, were they real? Or did I just dream of a cozy home and children and grandchildren who loved me? What has happened to my life's work? What do I keep forgetting? Where do I go from here? What am I supposed to do?

A certain itinerant resident, Robin, who recognizes no one here, walks the halls in a dignified fashion. She stopped me one day and said quite poignantly, "Do you know what they did to me? . . . I want to hold my mother so bad." I look down and slowly turn my head back and forth. Robin walks on.

Today she's still wandering around, haunted, wondering, looking for an answer that no one can give. With a blank expression she told a visitor in the lobby, "I've been dead for thirty years."

How do we know the difference between our dreams and waking reality? One way is consistency. We keep coming back to the same workaday world. Socially, we agree upon what is real and what is not, and those around us generally agree on the meaning of our daily experience. These two guideposts seem to dissolve in the case of our demented brothers and sisters. Imagine losing the distinction between dreaming and working. Imagine the logic of dreams permeating everyday life.

You don't have to be demented to suffer the loss of control while living here with us. Eva lives in her room with a minimum of help. She is basically "self-care." She voluntarily helps care for other residents during activities. She keeps her clothes in a padlocked closet. Yet one day when she spilled her tea, I saw this proud lady break down and cry like a baby, right there in the crowded dining hall, before God and everybody. It is the steady erosion of abilities that wears us down. Even our strongest residents constantly see their own near future in the diminished abilities of those around them. It's everywhere, within all of us, as persistent as Chinese water torture, eating away at who we think we are.

Midge is ninety-two, yet she believes that I am the first boy who ever kissed her. The naughty beau she remembers in me is a lad who plucked her cherry in the chicken yard, away from her mother's prying eyes.

When I get her up or lay her down, I move in close and I let her hug me. While she talks softly, her hand caresses my cheek or picks imaginary lint off my shirtsleeve. I give her a warm hug. Within a few seconds I feel her shoulder muscles relax. Her breathing slows. She chuckles, asks for a kiss, and tells me she loves me and asks me if I love her too. She tells me not to leave her and I give her my assurance. Occasionally I playfully refer to her tale about our first secret time together and how we kissed behind the barn and "made those old hens cackle all day."

Midge shared with a fellow aide, "I'm ninety-two, but I have a boyfriend." It may seem just playful to us, but to a lady like Midge I believe the false memory she creates fills in the holes that surround her days.

Our beautician, Liza, said that Midge came to her to ask to have her hair done because "my boyfriend is coming." This was the first time Midge had ever made such a request, so Liza asked Midge, "Who is your boyfriend." Midge said, "Tom, Tom, the piper's son, stole a goose and away he run."

When I gave Melka a bath one day she said, "Oh, boy, that's one for the books. A man giving a woman a bath. Haha!"

Paula also said in the shower, "Can you imagine finding a husband to do this for you? Oh, boy! If they could see me now." And as I was rinsing her off, "Do you want to have a couple of kids?"

"What do you mean?" I ask.

"Well, isn't it normal for a husband and wife to have kids?" Seeing my discomfort she lets me off the hook by saying with a laugh, "When the hell are we going to Paris, anyway?"

Barb's family came in for a visit one recent afternoon: her mother, her sister, and two young cousins. One cousin was crying. The whole troupe looked dejected and somber. I asked them what kind of personality Barb had before the accident that left her comatose. They said that she was a happy kid, "slow" but always wanting to help. I privately note that most twenty-seven-year-olds are not referred to as kids. They said that she was able to do some cross-stitching and she loved to listen to KTLS, her favorite pop radio station. To earn spending money, she cleaned the houses of several friends in the neighborhood. I see a photo of Barb in better days. I am surprised by how slender, trim, and affable she looked then.

The family visitors have taped a dozen greeting cards and sympathy cards on the wall opposite her bed. They also put up some family pictures grouped together in cutout frames. I asked if they had any video footage of Barb. It would help personalize our image of her while cleaning and tending her. The following week the father said that they had about ten seconds of Barb on video holding the baby at Christmas in front of the tree. Perhaps she was not the family member they were most proud to put in front of a camera.

It's apparent that she is very loved, though, perhaps even more so now after the accident. The tears and concern of the family are real. Care for her has consumed her father's life savings, I was told. But all this does not convince me that she truly resides here among the living.

Privately I wonder if Barb has gained a great deal more than we will ever know. Perhaps she is more alive now in some other reality not accessible to us. Perhaps she is dancing in Elysian fields or floating over soft horizons. But I keep such ruminations to myself. Whereas many people want to believe that she is here, I hope for her sake that she is not. How long will she be sentenced to stay with us?

In a moment of reflection, I wonder if the reason I do not see her consciously react, while others seem to, is because I don't want to look into the horror of her being trapped in a broken, shut-down body. I make a resolution to look more closely at that possibility. I will give Barb a chance.

Baths

Every day each aide has to give as many as five baths. Only a few residents actually like to be bathed. Marge, of course, routinely complains that she hasn't had a bath in months.

I gather up a fresh set of clothing and diapers, find the scheduled suspect, and roll him or her into an available shower room. The shower room is not the comfortable refuge that one might hope for. At home, I look forward to a chance to relax with a good book while luxuriating in a hot bath. Our shower room, by contrast, is a large clinical space with walls of glossy tan ceramic tiles and a gray, skid-resistant floor. When I first looked around this empty room, I found myself wondering, "Wow, do we have our own autopsy table in here?" It has an open shower stall, a huge whirlpool tub, and a toilet exposed and standing all alone in the corner. All of these appliances can be visually closed off by retractable curtains hanging in tracks from the suspended acoustic ceiling. The damp air has a heavy odor of disinfectant and feces, the product of routine accidents that do not always get completely hosed down.

Frequently I find that I have to leave a resident alone in the shower for a few moments to retrieve towels and washcloths or dispose of items littering the floor. Sometimes these items include neglected turds, because residents frequently defecate during their baths. This must be due in part to the open-bottom seating device. After a resident is stripped bare, he or she is seated on a shower chair made of white PVC plastic pipe fashioned basically into a toilet seat on wheels. This is the only practical arrangement that anyone can seem to come up with for washing people who are unable to stand. It is safe and convenient, but it does provoke an unfortunate evacuation reflex.

Showering also provides a good opportunity to check for impactions and various skin conditions. The resident sits in the shower chair situated over the floor drain. Then we lean over a knee-high wall designed to keep our feet from getting soaked. Using a hose with a sprinkler head and shampoo-bodywash from a gallon jug, we work up an ample lather. We wash under the folds of fat and flabby breasts and between mangled toes. We check for bruises, rashes, scrapes, skin tears, sores, abrasions, contusions, and fungus-infected toenails. The shower is usually over in five minutes unless the resident likes to luxuriate or happens to be fastidious. Drying also goes quickly. We clip toenails while they are still softened by the water. Many, perhaps most, residents have a fungus that makes their nails grow bulky and difficult to trim with a standard clipper.

Dressing residents with damp, tender skin while grappling with tight socks over damp and swollen feet can be a struggle. Walter, of course, is always a treat in the shower. "Get me outta here!" he bellows. "Dry me off!" "I said no, goddammit!" Even on the best days he cannot tolerate water on his bald pate. I out-flank him by positioning myself slightly to his rear, well outside his effective striking range. If he finds the chance, he grabs the shower hose and flings it over the knee wall with a hearty curse. Then, after all the struggling, as I begin to pat him dry, Walter ceremoniously bows his head and asks sweetly, "How much do I owe you, sir?"

On my very first day of work here I helped give Walter a shower. The maneuver required three people—one to wash him and two to restrain him by gripping a towel twisted around both wrists. At the time he looked like a rabid raccoon. Deep-purple bruises from a bad fall and two black eyes had transformed his face into a primitive war mask. He was cursing and fighting with all his might. Aides were laughing and dodging, not out of ridicule, I believe, but out of participation in his vigorous spirit.

But times change, old warriors fade away. Lately I am able to bathe him by myself. I arm myself with graham crackers and require help only during the finale—lifting him back onto his wheelchair while drying his backside and pulling up diapers and sweatpants. Walter's knees collapse after about ten seconds when he attempts to stand.

I walked into work recently (I usually clock in before 5 A.M.) and there was Chester sitting in the vestibule holding a lawn chair upside down over his head. "What's up, Chester?" I asked.

"Ceiling's going to fall in, you'll see." Within five minutes he heard a tornado looming directly overhead, then the approach of Russian bombers, and finally the return of the Blitzkrieg over London as well as the shelling of Corregidor.

Another day, Chester came out from his room in sweatpants, bare-chested and trying with some difficulty to pull a shirt on over his head. I moved in to help him. I soon discovered that he had his arms in a second set of sweatpants. I pointed this out, and Chester chuckled and shuffled off to his room.

Chester tells stories of discovering half a million dollars in gold that was hijacked and stashed by the Japanese somewhere in Luzon, just north of Manila. He won't tell me exactly where. He says he has a metal plate in his head that makes him magnetic. He jokes that on his wedding night his pristine nubile wife asked if he could "please soften it up a little. It seems too hard." His laugh is infectious. When he greets me in the hall I ask him how it's going, and Chester will hold up his thumb and forefinger about two inches apart and say, "Oh, about like that," while laughing, covertly referring to the current status of his proudest appendage.

Chester's doctor documents his condition as "amiably and pleasantly confused." He almost always rises before 5 A.M. One morning, though, when I was sent to get him up, I had a surprisingly difficult time rousing him. Then a nurse casually mentioned that he had gone over to another nursing home to visit his wife. Their romantic interlude the night before explained why I could not get him up that morning. They have a happy marriage and used to live together here, but someone (I don't know who) decided they had to be separated. The problem is that his wife is apparently oversexed. She depleted Chester's stamina sufficiently that he started losing weight. As I stated, in our system we cannot tolerate weight loss, even for the happiest of reasons. I could think of worse ways to go.

This is what I love about these folks in decline, particularly the demented souls among them: they lack discrimination in love. They have lost all their social chips. They couldn't care less if I am rich or handsome or beautiful. They only see what I do in my own free-form style. They allow me the privilege of letting my heart flow as freely as I like. This is the only group of people that I have found who live up to Martin Luther King's vision—they judge people by the "content of their character," or, more accurately, by the moral quality of their actions.

I love it when they disregard my personal space. They feel free to move right in, as free as a small child sitting on Grandpa's lap rooting through his shirt pocket or poking around, inspecting the features of his nose and lips. These old people freshen me up a bit.

Play does not flow uninterrupted, however. I watch this job wear me down physically and emotionally. Our moods swing here as they do everywhere else, only much more abruptly, and politeness among staffers goes right out the window in such a raw atmosphere. It's sometimes hard to pretend everything is rosy and proper while scooping up shit.

Life Goes On

I am trying to show you what life is like here by taking a snapshot. It is a group portrait, a collage of people thrown together by happenstance, captured with a wide lens and shallow depth of focus. Even at their moribund pace, however, our residents will not stand still long enough for me to take a picture without someone's clear image bleeding into a blur. I come home from work and jot down a few lines. Naturally I pick out salient features and memorable anecdotes. I alter individual stories to fit the general picture, to protect privacy, and to create more flow. There is no plot or character development to speak of. Long-term care just rambles on without clear purpose or direction. So if you, the reader, are trying to keep all the characters straight, it's probably a waste of effort. In the short course of writing this book, many of our residents died or went home and were replaced by new residents.

It may seem at first glance that nothing much happens in a nursing home, but this place is a cascade of lives in free fall. Mundane occurrences are barely events at all, compared with "regular" life, but the big stuff here, the major life events, assault our elders at a frightening pace.

I also watch the effect this place has on me. I see myself becoming much more emotionally expressive as a result of working with my old friends. It's because these people are so safe. Their emotions become as transparent as their skin.

Skooter died and now Gilda and Lucy occupy his room. Skooter caught pneumonia. The doctor diagnosed it on my day off. He was hospitalized very briefly and then within the hour he died. He was a good man, but I have no sense of missing him. One comes to expect death and, with a few exceptions, usually not make much of a fuss over it. Or perhaps I've just used up all of my grief.

Gilda looks relatively young, probably less than seventy. She is a stroke victim, heavy set and wheelchair bound. She broke her hip and suffered a debilitating stroke while lying sedated on the operating table. Her right foot is totally limp. She is not much of a bother, except that she is incontinent and a prodigious urinator. Her urine has the most acrid odor imaginable. She gives the impression of being quite neurotic. Gilda does not hold conversations, but she will answer direct questions rather clearly. I potty her right after breakfast as soon as I get a chance. If I am lucky I get to reload her panty liner before her pants show a wet spot. Often she reaches out and says to me, "I'm scared."

"What are you afraid of?" I ask.

"I don't know. Please help me. I'm scared. Please help me."

I try to comfort her but have no idea what monsters lurk within her. I let her hug me, I pat her shoulder, I tell her that her days of worrying are over and that everything she needs is free for her right here. None of my words have a discernible effect on her anxiety. Perhaps she could use more potent psychoactive drugs. She just won't be comforted. When she holds my hand she is loath to let me go. Lately when Gilda pleads, "Please help me, I'm so scared," I respond with "I'm scared too, Gilda. We're all scared here, every one of us." And it seems to help somewhat, if only momentarily. Her life is fear.

Gilda spends her mornings sitting in her wheelchair just outside her room. She lists slightly to the right and seems to take no particular interest in any kind of activity or diversion. Twice I have coaxed her to let me roll her out into our courtyard, where she can breathe some fresh air and look at the hills in the distance. She agrees, but hesitantly. She feels safer in her spot in the hall, where she can poise like a mouse just barely poking its jittery nose out of its hole, always ready to dart back into safety. Age has not softened her fears, instead it has eroded her defenses.

I try not to get irritated with her for being such a heavy lift and having to be pottied so often, which really may be a way of saying I am disappointed in myself for not being able to reach behind her fears. I give her a quick peck on the cheek and meet a stubble of bristly white whiskers.

Gilda's roommate, Lucy, is ninety-four and totally independent. She has a deep scowl permanently etched into her face. I know that she was an Iowa farmer's wife. Nevertheless she rises as late as possible. Maybe the roosters on her farm worked the second shift. She prowls the halls all night, looking for I don't know what, possibly a hole in the fence. Even at the height of summer she keeps the room heater running on full blast. Add to that multiple layers of blankets, sweaters, scarves, and afghans, and she does just fine, thank you very much.

On her first morning with us I went to her closet and selected an outfit, just as I would do with any resident. Lucy rejected the blouse I'd selected. She rejected the next four blouses I selected. Finally I coaxed her into her wheelchair and put her in front of her closet and asked her which outfit she wanted to wear. "I'm not going to tell you," she said flatly. Immediately my estimation of her character skyrocketed. I have learned to respect her space and to leave her to her own devices as much as possible.

I was advised to turn Lucy's TV on and crank up the volume to rouse her from her deep slumber. But I prefer, instead, to take a few seconds to just sit beside her on the edge of her bed and stroke and massage her hand and tell her she's just going to have to get up: "The cows need milking." Lucy responds by softly agreeing in a puff of stale breath that could pickle a Bantam rooster, "Well, okay, I guess." She has an old photo of herself as a young woman pinned to the wall among some thirty-odd pictures of cats playing with skeins of yarn and teasing lizards to death on the cement patio. An old photo of her as a teen shows the very same down-turned mouth and frown she sports today. I unpin it for a moment and show it to her. "I always was serious," she notes.

Lucy spends quite a long time alone in her bathroom. One time she left the door ajar and announced that she needed a washbasin. So I ran around and finally scrounged up a plastic Rubbermaid dish tub for her. She looked at me as though I was nuts and with emphasis repeated her need for a washbasin. Fortunately a more savvy coworker came by and interceded. She went directly to the linen cart and brought Lucy the washcloth, which is what she really wanted. Days later, when Lucy insisted that she needed a raincoat (it was raining outside), my coworker knew enough to reach directly for her sweater, and she was perfectly satisfied.

With time one gets better at deciphering approximations of meanings. Once while I, in my scrubs, was fixing her bed with its five blankets and an afghan, she asked me, "Are you the angel?"

"No," I said, "the doctor will be in later."

"Do you lay down anywhere?"

"I have a house fifteen minutes down the road from here," I replied.

Her daughter, Rhea, came to visit. After a few seconds I saw that Rhea's countenance is every bit as serious as her mother's. I surmise by her expression that Rhea is none too anxious to be pleased by nursing-home reality. In general, family members seem to be either very kind to us or the exact opposite. In Rhea's case, I find that my first impression was defensive and totally wrong. Over time I have come to know her as considerate and kind.

Why am I staying with this kind of work? Inertia perhaps. "I get mad as hell at you for keeping this shitty job," Marge tells me. "I wouldn't do what you do for anybody. You could do way better than this, in a minute. You're too intelligent for this kind of work. I told Marty you weren't coming back after your days off. You're making a damned liar out of me."

"What'll you do when I quit?"

With a smile behind her growl she said, "Well, I'll get mad at you for quitting, I guess."

Youth is not necessarily the most beautiful stage in life. Character creates its own ambiance. I have an old oak tree in my front yard. It caught a disease and over the course of a few years, it gradually died, branch by branch, limb by limb. Twigs went bare and dropped off, then branches stood out alone, stiff and abandoned by foliage. I trimmed off arterial branches because they posed a vague threat of falling on a car, but I left as much as I could. A wisteria vine invited itself into the fresh openings and climbed for sunlight. Oak bark fell to the ground in curled sheets.

The main trunk still stands, a huge post with bare knuckles covered with a lovely vine. All of these final, sad stages appeared to me to contain their own beauty. The death and decay were not ugly. The invasion of parasites and insects brought in welcome visits from a family of pileated woodpeckers.

I could have cut that oak down when I knew that its health was lost. I would have gained a little bit more lawn to mow, but I'm certainly glad that I didn't. If we can see the beauty of age in a tree, why can't we see it in our own skin?

When a dietary aide teased me by saying I was getting a bald spot on the top of my head, I nearly panicked and ran to the closest mirror to check it out.

Old people are certainly not bland. Time imprints character in the wrinkles and folds of age-worn flesh. Pasty, sagging, craggy imperfections, wild idiosyncrasies and demented cravings, all work together to form a deeply human tapestry. But a beautiful person does not always wear beautiful skin. Often the opposite is true.

Of course Miss America is a beauty. But does her beauty affect me personally? Not at all. We are separated by her beauty. However, when I come across a person who is wholly alive and free, who shares a moment of full attention, I sense a shift, recognizing the beauty of who we both are. We both feel more free and precious.

That is another kind of beauty, the kind that grows rather than fades.

Interactions

We cannot directly enter the mental landscapes that our demented residents somehow meld in their conversations. The demented seem to make sense to each other often without using any recognizable language. We have a coven of Alzheimer's ladies who habitually congregate near the water cooler or drift about holding hands and practicing the social graces you might find in a delightful playground tea party. Old men seem more solitary, but our women love to party. Many, I suspect, simply enjoy belonging to a group even while playing a form of social solitaire. Perhaps it's like the first day of preschool. They don't really know each other, but they like to feel included, so they move together in a friendly orbit. Conversations in this klatch are typically devoid of meaningful content, just bits and fragments of free-floating niceties, parallel monologues, and non sequiturs. Not all that different, now that I come to think of it, from the way I hear some of my neighbors talk.

Occasionally residents who formerly led lives of propriety, reserve, and kindness enter our facility and, to the horror of sons and daughters, are transformed into foul-mouthed, hostile, and rude sociopaths. I suspect that they have long repressed dark feelings and ill-mannered sentiments. Dementia pops the lid off moral restrictions. Native innocence reemerges and freedom flowers.

The spirit that the rest of us harbor is really not so unlike that of people here—we just don't like to let it out. Our residents carry the full range of human emotions and often display them quite openly. When you have lost everything including your ego, you have little fear of honesty.

On the other hand, many residents only want to sleep. A resident like Barb represents the vegetative extreme—I still am not convinced she ever has a conscious thought. I have gone back and spent more time with her, talked to her, and looked for signs of awareness, but I still conclude we aides are just maintaining a body with her name on it. The range of behaviors in long-term care is quite broad. The residents' movements are visibly slow, and their sense of direction seems blurry and confused, but what passionate dramas remain hidden from our eyes?

Gracie likes to help Midge. Recently the two of them apparently held a discussion in their room about walkers. Gracie offered Midge the use of one of her walkers. (She collects them in her room—we're not sure where she snatches them from.) Midge thought it might be fun to take one out for a spin. She got herself up out of bed, which is rather rare, and promptly fell down. From out in the hall we heard peals of laughter coming from their room. They both thought her fall was hilarious.

Later the joy went out of Midge's misadventure. She'd bruised a rib in her fall, which brought on three days of "Please, God, let me die!" ad nauseam. "Take me to the end of the road and let me die there," she told me. Then a second later, with eyes wide open and alarmed, "You won't leave me alone there, will you?"

Recently, when Midge had one of her regular bowel blowouts, Gracie took it upon herself to strip Midge's soiled bed linens. Often Gracie will neatly fold the blankets and sheets that Midge would otherwise keep in an unsatisfying jumble.

Audrey scrapes her neighbor's dishes after lunch. Vela spoon-feeds Melka when she's too sleepy to feed herself. We all need a purpose to fill our days satisfactorily, or perhaps the kinetic memories of past service are so ingrained in the muscles themselves that the motions continue long after the lights in the control tower go dim.

Paula sits in her wheelchair just outside her room, looking bored, scowling. When anyone approaches her with a greeting she either perks up for the moment or comes back with a sarcastic comment. I pass by her chair countless times in a day's work. Occasionally I bend down and give her a quick peck on the cheek, but most often I breeze on by. One day she said, almost in tears, "I was afraid you were mad at me." So I knelt down beside her chair and spent a few moments visiting with her. Sometime later, as I gave her a pat on the shoulder more or less in passing, she said, "Hey! Do I have a husband or a traveling salesman?" Potato chips are her favorite diversion. We can usually pacify her with a handful of chips on a napkin. But Paula cannot turn around in her wheelchair, and she worries about what Betty might be up to behind her back in their room. The threat of her roommate just out of view etches a constant frown across Paula's brow.

Meanwhile, Betty is preoccupied with changing clothes or packing up to "go to Indianapolis," and she fears that she's going to soil herself and worries that Kent is about to divorce her. On lucky days, Betty might get a manicure and a nail polishing from Activities, and all will be well while she is receiving attention and getting dolled up. One day Betty laid claim to a loaded ice chest that was left sitting on a cart in the hall. (We use a regular ice cooler, similar to the kind you might take to a tailgate party, to restock the rooms with ice.) Betty was convinced that her husband was buried under the ice and would not be deterred from her search.

Roxy passes Mariah in the hall. Suddenly she is convinced that Mariah is her mother. She coos and lathers Mariah with abundant love. Mariah accepts her adulation. Roxy bobs her hair with a hand behind the ear and says, "Oh, I'm sorry you have to see me like this, I must look terrible."

Solitary Lola eats packets of diet sugar or sleeps. In the midst of any crowd she remains alone.

Melka approaches Melanie and asks, "What time is it?" Melanie, a retired elementary school teacher, with perfectly erect posture and precise, exaggerated diction, echoes in a singsong, "What time is it?"

Melka tries again. "What time is it?"

Melanie replies musically, eyes wide open, smiling broadly at open space, "What time is it?"

Melka again: "What time is it?"

Melanie: "What time is it?"

Melka, getting irritated: "Didn't you go to school?"

Melanie, innocently: "Didn't you go to school?"

Melka gives up. "Are you some kind of idiot?"

Melanie faithfully echoes, "Are you some kind of idiot?"

Melka throws her hands down disgusted. Melanie holds her smile, unaffected.

Ivy reads about Elvis and Princess Di in her *National Enquirer* and Marge extorts a ride back and forth from her perch next to Marty to her room to watch the soaps on channel 10 or rummage through the snacks in her dresser. Marge will say, "Tom, take me back to my room for a drink of ice water." Then while she has me captive she needs to potty, to wash her hands, to eat a snack, to adjust the curtains, to turn up the heat, to get a tissue, to adjust the exact position of her remote control. Marge is bored beyond tears.

Marge looks forward to watching *Dr. Quinn, Medicine*

Woman every Saturday, as long as its on channel 10. When the same show appears on channel 3 she won't have anything to do with it. Our seniors are great for brand loyalty and routine.

We have a large activities room with a big-screen TV and rows of folding Masonite tables for playing games of the sort you are likely to find in a church basement. Bingo, Wednesdays at 2:30, is by far the most popular activity. The fans are fully engaged gamblers. Typical prize money is twenty-five cents per game, but it can go all the way up to a dollar if you "black out." The games are easily rigged by allowing residents to keep their partially filled cards from one game to the next, so every player gets more than an even chance to become a winner. Even folks like Zelda, with perfectly lucid minds, get hooked on Bingo, the black hole of boredom. Slot machines and video poker would do very well here.

Some residents have lately taken to crayons and coloring books. Our more fastidious ladies can sit for hours, staying neatly inside the lines. Some are given towels to fold. One or two cannot help cleaning up dirty dishes at various tables following a food-related activity, or scraping food scraps together into a colorful soup, or stacking plates and cups together in messy and satisfyingly creative patterns.

At ten o'clock nearly every morning Lois, the activity director, leads residents through a half-hour routine of exercises. They sit in a grand oval, wave their arms about, sing the hokey-pokey, then eat the greasy donuts that Lois passes out.

Another popular activity is balloon swatting, where residents sit in a big circle and use fly swatters to bat inflated balloons. This simple, easily controlled combat frequently brings uncommunicative residents back to life for a few minutes. It's an easy gross motor exercise and produces lots of smiles.

Other attempts are not as satisfying. Residents are given a certain time slot to "reminisce" about preselected topics, which often seems to flop. Perhaps it's a bit too staged and artificial. Nostalgia is big in the conventional wisdom of how to entertain seniors.

Activities staff also read aloud to assembled groups of residents. Perhaps the facilitator herself gets bored. We see a lot of white heads nodding off. Which, now that I think about it, may be the point.

Kindhearted volunteers occasionally call upon us with microphone and amplifier to preach or lead sing-alongs. Typically the audience response is nearly catatonic. The range of talent among guest performers is fantastic—from the gifted and disciplined to the truly afflicted. We provide a tough, if not discriminating, audience.

Once a week Lois rents an inoffensive and sentimental "family values" movie and shows it on the big-screen TV. This movie could be confused with any other movie concurrently showing on our various cable channels, except for the dimming of room lights and the popcorn.

The activity room has a large bulletin board covered with red and blue display paper and, in cutout letters, the words "Resident of the Month." The bulletin board is attached to the wall at a standard height—which means that for practical purposes it is useless for most of our residents, who are wheelchair bound and suffer from poor vision. Currently the Resident of the Month is Patrick, a long-term denizen of the back hall. Patrick is among the least presentable of our residents. He spends his days and nights curled in a compact ball, his knees fixed almost at eye level. His feet will move no more than two or three inches from his atrophied buttocks. Both of his arms are drawn up tight against his chest. His fingers and toes flare out in various and unexpected directions. Patrick is unable to make any sound other than a single note he hoots or howls. He is, however, blessed with a devout and loving wife, Nell. She comes by quite regularly, smiling, slowly hobbling on her cane, to feed him and check on his condition. She sews open-at-the-back shirts for him. She mends and alters clothing of other residents out of the goodness of her heart. These split-backed shirts comprise Patrick's entire wardrobe, besides a light blanket to cover his knees and bottom. Nell alone seems able to decipher his meaning (beyond the obvious extremes of anger or pleasure). None of us doubt her authority in this matter.

The Resident of the Month display features a list of Patrick's favorite colors and activities (gardening and travel—"I want to go to Yellowstone," it says under his name) and several family photos. Among them is a formal photograph taken in 1936. It shows Patrick as a dashing young man in a stylish fedora, padded suit, and tie. Nell says that he was so handsome, with "spectacular muscles" from working in an open-hearth steel mill. "He was very active," she says with a smile that is meant to convey a world of meaning.

I have only known the ninety-pound shell of this man, and I am shocked to see him shown in his former prowess. I cannot fathom his present reality. Does he remember himself? I asked Nell if she thinks he remembers his life or knows what's going on. She doubts that he does. I am amazed that these two extremes can be made to fit within the frame of a single life. How is it possible for one and the same person to be young and beautiful one moment and a literal basket case the next? Is he the same man?

I shudder.

Late Shift

For a month I moved my schedule to the second shift—from 3 to 11 P.M. Thought I'd give it a shot. The evening shift is quieter. We have only one meal to deal with. It's much easier to feed residents a light evening meal and then let them retire at their leisure. By comparison, the first shift is a constant bustle. On days, I almost never take a break. On evenings, there is plenty of time to visit. Days are filled with tension, evenings are much more peaceful.

Everyone attributes this collective sigh to the top staff—they all go home. An air of tranquility settles over the hall when the folks in dry-cleaned clothing finally leave the building. It's a variation on the trickle-down effect. Even though the administrators and other top staff mostly stay in their offices, their presence is still felt by nurses, and their tension flows downhill to us. Generally upper echelons are polite and competent people, but they too work under pressure and tend to find little time or cause to interact with us. I notice that as the law relaxes, a greater common sense reemerges in the after-hours. During the day shift, everyone toes the line, ostensibly going by the rules, living under fear of censure. But by the time the sun sets, a greater peacefulness fills the air. Even our hard-nosed nurses relax noticeably as the office lights dim.

And besides all this, it's a relief to get away from the demand of my regular residents on 300 Hall, demands which I have helped create by being such a spoiler. The charge nurse assigns me to a back hall. I don't know the habits of these residents, so I become inefficient all over again. On the plus side, though, these back hall residents don't expect much of anything from me.

The only new reality unique to evenings is Sundowner's syndrome, which is a term that we use loosely to describe some people who may be pleasantly confused during the day but transform into the unpleasantly confused and combative as the sun goes down. I have seen a few of our most endearing ladies suddenly turn into veritable vampires and werewolves of the night. Audrey, who loves to cuddle and mother all of us during the day, can suddenly turn violent and claw at our eyes as the sun sets. We have some night stalkers and several insomniacs who just roam up and down the dark halls, which usually are, to my relief, quiet and empty.

I answered Selina's call light one evening at about 9 P.M. She borrowed my ear to rant about her bed, how it had not been properly made all day: the bedspread was almost touching the floor. She complained about her roommate. Earlier in the day Mimi sat in Selina's soft chair and moved her water pitcher. Selina wanted to know why she couldn't get a decent roommate and why she had to put up with our neglect.

Finally, she lay herself down in bed. I sat down in her wheelchair and positioned myself beside her. Without saying a word, I simply held Selina's hand. In a few seconds Selina was crying.

"I'm so alone. I don't know what I'm going to do. I can't do anything these days, my hip hurts me so bad, especially when I stand. It's the cancer, ya know. I've worked hard all my life. I clerked in stores, I worked in restaurants, I took care a babies. Now I can't even baby-sit. I can't run after the young'ns, ya know?

What am I gonna do? Ah, I guess I'll be all right with Jesus takin' care a me. I figure I'll be all right. Yeah, I'll be all right."

I had nothing to add to her soliloquy. After a few moments her eyes closed softly and I silently left.

We have an unusually compelling couple that comes together every evening. Lester is in his mid-eighties and stone deaf. He cares for himself, reads newspapers and works crossword puzzles throughout the day. Then, after the evening meal, Lester rolls himself down to the back hall and finds his friend, Nora. Nora is immobile and, we suppose, demented. She cannot talk or move, though her eyes radiate alertness and joy. Sometimes she smiles and makes musical cooing sounds. Sometimes she laughs softly for no apparent reason. She sits in her wheelchair with her legs raised on extended foot pedals. Surely it's her unrelenting contentment and profound happiness that convince us that she must be out of her mind.

Lester rolls his chair close to Nora's and puts his arm around her. He holds her in this position for about an hour, every night without fail. He simply sits there, holding her. She smiles.

It seems that years ago Lester and Nora were neighbors— nothing more, just friendly neighbors. As time progressed they were both widowed and independently became residents at a neighboring nursing home. There they found solace in each other's company. Nora's family objected, thinking that even platonic romance showed disrespect for the memory of Nora's deceased husband. So they moved her out and over to our facility to protect her from Lester's affection. Then Lester just followed her here.

They make a lovely couple. At first Nora's family members asked that we put her to bed early, to discourage such a public display of affection. One of our nurses also found this overt behavior offensive and put forward efforts to separate them. That nurse is no longer with us, thank God. No one bothers them anymore. They've become a fixture here, a small sanctuary of the evening's twilight hour.

Similarly, an aide approached me with some urgency in her voice and said, "We need to have a talk."

"Okay."

"Are you aware that there are women on this hall who are in love with you? I mean really in love with you?"

"Uh-huh."

"Do you know that Paula thinks you are her husband? I mean, do you encourage her to believe that?"

"I show her all the affection I can. Yeah, sure I let her believe whatever she wants. So what? I don't put those ideas in her head, but I don't interfere with her fancies, either. That's just her. I tell her I only work here, but she lets that slide by. Sure I encourage her to feel that I belong to her. So what if she thinks that we go way back together?

"I just give them my full attention and they can put that wherever they want to in their minds. Gracie turned me into her stepson for a short while. One time at lunch Gilda lit up when she recognized me as her grade-school teacher. So what are you afraid might happen?"

"Well, I don't know exactly. I just wanted to make sure you were aware of what's going on."

"Lea thought I was her fiancé for months. She followed me around the halls every day. After a while she finally figured out that nothing was going to come of it, and it just dropped off. This happens all the time."

I spent some extra time with Barb, looking for signs of a meaningful inner life and not finding it. Again I concluded that she's just not here among us. I wonder why this had to happen to her. What does it mean to keep her here among us? What can she be contributing or gaining from being with us? Then by chance I came across Karon, on the night shift, too, as she was tending to Barb. Barb is Karon's pet resident. I peered inside for a moment before Karon noticed me.

Karon finds time to come in to shampoo Barb's hair and priss her up, even though these and other tasks are scheduled for the day shift. In that room, I could feel Karon's love for Barb. It wasn't in anything Karon said or did as much as in her extraordinarily soft and tender manner. Karon, a loving, lonely soul who just can't trust adults, finds safe refuge in Barb's misfortune.

At that moment I recognized that perhaps Barb as she is today has a reason for being here, a real function, a usefulness, and not for Karon alone. Perhaps Barb's role for us is as a love object. She is just someone to love. Barb comes with this guarantee: "I will never hurt or frighten you, I will never disappoint you, I will never snap back at you or send you away." Loving Barb is entirely safe, and maybe we need that.

Harold celebrated his ninety-seventh birthday. About twenty family members came in from three surrounding states. There was a barbecue and great salads made with extra-virgin olive oil and artichoke hearts, and two nicely decorated cakes from the Wal-Mart bakery. There were festive mylar helium balloons and many candles. Long tables were arranged in a U shape that took up the entire activity room. Zelda was seated at the head of the table. Harold sat off to the side in his recliner. The eldest son tapped the side of a champagne glass with his fork and called for silence. Then he led the extended family in an inspired group prayer and an invocation of filial piety. Harold calmly and gracefully accepted all the attention and adulation. Then he ate his standard dietary fare of pureed meat with mashed potatoes and carrots. Harold's children invited me to join in the fun. I ate Polish sausage on a bun and some fine salad and accepted their sincere gratitude for caring for Harold.

Harold stayed sitting up in a soft chair for a full five hours. He was alert and attentive throughout. I would not have guessed that Harold could find that much stamina within him. Affection abounded, great-grandkids fussed with each other and ran around Harold's La-Z-Boy in bounding circles.

Harold extinguished his own candles. It remained unspoken, but everyone came to this celebration to recognize Harold's grand finale. All in all, it was a job well done.

Marge ignited a donnybrook with her nurse last evening. It took place in her bathroom. Marge normally brushes her own teeth before bed, holding her brush in her curled fist, then swishing out her mouth with Listerine as part of her nightly ritual. Her Listerine supply had run out, but she also possesses a bottle of hydrogen peroxide to use instead. So she decided to swish out with that. Her nurse, Cheryl, said, "I just can't let you keep this in here, but I'll pour out some in a paper cup and let you use it one dose at a time."

Marge instantly became livid. Her mouth screwed into a snarl and she barked, "What the hell are you talking about? That's my bottle and I'll do whatever the hell I want with it. Get your ass out of my face! *Now!*" She was flushed and shaking with fury.

Cheryl calmly stood her ground. "Marge, I can't just leave this bottle in here. If you did something with it and hurt yourself, I'd get in trouble for it. Now just let me pour out a little for you to use now . . ."

"*No*, goddammit! I don't want any of it now. Get the hell out of here this very minute!"

Cheryl softly repeated her offer to let Marge have a single dose.

"No! That's my bottle and I've been using that stuff for years. My doctor had me using it when I had a bad ear. And I used it for my teeth lots of times before."

Later that shift after Marge was safely tucked in bed, Cheryl gave me the bottle and told me to put it above her bathroom cabinet, out of Marge's reach. I told Cheryl that Marge got so angry because she was afraid of losing control of even small details of her own life. Cheryl agreed. I asked her if she really was afraid that she would hurt herself somehow with the peroxide.

"No," she replied, "it's just the idea of leaving it in the room."

I do not know what that reply meant. What idea? I suspect that Cheryl is in the habit of protecting herself from possible incrimination regardless of how remote. She admitted that the chance of any real danger was practically zero.

I surmise that the threat of malpractice is by far more central to our operation than the residents' control over their own lives and property. "Safety first" means safety from lawsuits; caring for oneself, independence, and self-esteem matter less.

As for her part in the exchange, Marge got to fortify the walls of her anger. She was able to blame her problems on something outside her control: "This damned place is the cause of all my problems."

On the following day, Marge bragged to me about how she told "that nurse" just exactly what she thought of her. "I hope I didn't scare you," she said. "Now you can see how mad I can get."

Her sense of pride in her anger was unmistakable. She acted like a dominant gorilla beating the ground with a tree trunk. At heart, Marge is a garden-variety terrorist. She would mold her world by the strictures of her anger. Despite her affection for me, I thank God she holds no real power.

Luna was moved to a back hall for her own protection. Luna's daughter tired of retrieving her mother's necklaces and perfume from Joan, her kleptomaniac roommate. For more than a week Luna compared every aide back there to me. I received a certain amount of ribbing about that from my coworkers, which I took as a grudging compliment.

As a result, I notice that now I treat Luna with even more patience and kindness simply because she has nurtured a flattering affection for me. The flip side of that, of course, is that she is incompetent. So what is the meaning of her affection? It feels real enough, but I have no idea if she knows who I am at all. I may remind her of someone in her idealized past.

Now when I interact with Luna, I am careful not to tell her who I am, relying on her extremely poor eyesight to release me and let my affections become more generalized in her mind.

The situation with Luna also makes me wonder about being more careful with my affections in general. Another example: Betty has begun to worry that her husband will find out that she likes me. One day Betty said she saw a "big nigger down the hall looking at me." Then she added, "I would never marry a big nigger, but I would marry you."

I have stopped kissing her on the cheek. Now I act a bit more formal with Betty. I do not want to add fuel to her fear. She has often talked about being beaten by drunken parents and being placed in a "guardian home" as a child. Some days, she packs up a few articles of clothing and asks the way to the "Indiana State Prison where my husband is being kept for beating up Biff," her son.

Luna's bed is now occupied by a new resident, Roxy, who is somewhat demented and very hard of hearing. She is a friendly character with a wonderful Texas drawl and a floppy set of dentures. She is fairly easy to care for, since she is usually continent and prefers to sit alone in her room and look out the window.

She was suspicious of me when she first arrived. She told her daughter that I was an intruder who jumped up and down on her bed. After a short period of increasing exposure she has come to trust me. Roxy told me, "It's hard to be in a strange town with no friends and your daughter saying you're crazy."

She gets on her roommate Joan's case, calling her "fat and lazy." In truth, Joan's not all that fat. From the start, Roxy ragged on Joan for "not paying her share of the rent." After being with us for about a week she said, "Ten months you've been here with me and you haven't paid me any rent, not one red cent." Joan rolls over in bed and faces the wall, not saying anything.

Like so many residents, Roxy is worried about her money. She wanted me to call the FBI about her social security check turning up missing. I had our bookkeeper write her a receipt for the money that her daughter had signed over to the facility, but then Roxy kept trying to cash in the receipt.

Roxy used to be an antique furniture dealer. One day she looked out her window and saw a memorial service being held on the lawn. It was our ceremony to honor the memory of residents who died in the previous year. Well-dressed family members were sitting in rows of lawn chairs with their backs to Roxy and facing a man in a black cassock holding up a chalice. Roxy perked up and said she wanted to "hurry up and go to that auction out there."

Last night at about ten o'clock, Beula got herself out of bed and started to patrol the halls. She dressed herself in a well-coordinated outfit and combed her hair smartly. She put herself in her wheelchair and then started to pull herself along the long handrails. I mention this because Beula routinely becomes pathetically unable to do anything for herself when it's time to get moving. She dresses haphazardly and moans pitifully at the slightest motion. Throughout the day she'll raise her hand to flag down any available Samaritan and say, "Please help me," as though it took every last scintilla of her energy just to get those self-pitying words out. Normally we tend to ignore her requests in favor of other residents with more pressing needs.

As it happened, last night I had little to do when I found myself in her presence, so I knelt before her and asked her some questions. Immediately I saw her pitiful face light up. Someone was paying attention to her. Over and over I have to learn this same lesson: there is an interesting person on the other side of all the problems and misery. It turns out that Beula was married for twenty-six years to another of our residents, Bill. Bill worked as an upper-level administrator for the federal prison system. Together the two of them lived next to the warden's mansion on Alcatraz Island, one of the most dramatic and beautiful sites in America. She once met the Birdman of Alcatraz. This introduction transformed Beula for me. Within two minutes, she transformed from a problem to be dealt with into a real person with a fascinating past.

I had a similar experience when, on my way out, I dropped in on Zelda and Harold. Zelda was already in bed. She reached her arms out and invited me over. I leaned down and kissed her cheek as she hugged me warmly and patted my back. "How come I never get to see you anymore?" she asked. I gave the usual excuse. For several minutes I sat on the edge of her bed as we chatted quietly in the subdued light. We made small talk. We discussed and compared the string of head nurses that Zelda and I have witnessed parade through the home. I enjoyed this visit with Zelda, much more than I enjoy serving her. Somehow, serving her feels burdensome. I am pleased to be her chosen friend, but I feel degraded as the instrument that makes her world order much tidier than my own will ever be. She puts herself above me.

Back on Days

In our sleep
Pain, which cannot forget,
Falls drop by drop upon the heart until,
In our own despair, against our will,
Comes wisdom, through the awful grace of God.
—Aeschylus

I received a call on my answering machine asking me to come in to work early. It seems that only one aide out of the six who were scheduled bothered to show up for work. Five no-call-no-shows left one aide and two nurses in care of 124 residents. We need more than that just to satisfy the fire code. I went in early to help get people up. I felt tired and resentful on the way in to work.

When I found Ro in bed, she'd already had two episodes of diarrhea; this was her third in a few hours. I moved her to the shower room to wash her off. As I seated her on the toilet near the whirlpool, she said lethargically, "I feel sick," and quietly went limp and then totally unresponsive. She could not keep her eyes open. She leaned to one side and began to drool. Her skin became bluish, cool, and clammy. I summoned two nurses who rushed in to check her out. We had to look in her chart to see if she had a code (emergency instructions on whether to give her CPR or not). Her chart stipulated, "Only revive if you think she'll come back." We pondered the prophetic implications for a few seconds, shrugged, and then proceeded to do what we could for her. When in doubt, err on the side of caution. The pulse ox (a gadget to measure heart beat and blood oxygen) failed to work. Our stethoscope fell apart in the nurse's hands. We put Ro on oxygen and sent her off in an ambulance. The consensus was that she must have had either a heart attack or a stroke. The hospital report came in later: septic urinary tract infection.

Right after breakfast, Aldo threw a psychotic fit with fantastic energy and vigor. Aldo is a retired nursing-home accountant, a dapper dresser and at times a pleasure to banter with (if his laconic quips and spontaneous laughter can be called banter). "Aldo, do you want to take a bath?" I asked once. "It would be an honor!" was his catch-all reply. But not yesterday. Suddenly he became frenetic in his chair, even stood up (I had never seen him stand before), and shouted obscenities and non sequiturs. As he winced and gnashed his teeth, he put all of his might into uncoordinated kicks, shoves, and wrangles as if he were trying to throw an invisible steer in a phantom rodeo. I turned his wheelchair handgrips against the handrail so that his kicks would only propel him closer to the wall. Then I and another aide held his arms tightly in place while a nurse gave him a shot of Ativan, a tranquilizer. We still had to hold him down for perhaps fifteen minutes until he gradually lost strength as the drug took effect.

Meanwhile, dainty and demented little Jolene walked up smiling brightly, and Aldo managed to land a kick on her thigh. Jolene was knocked back a bit but nonetheless continued to talk happy gibberish at Aldo; gingerly, she approached him again, as if she'd just found in this meat grinder a long lost friend. A third aide came by and led Jolene away.

All of this commotion took place a couple of yards from Harold and Zelda's room. Zelda was waiting at her doorway in full view of this ruckus. Nonetheless, she sent word down my way that she needed to go to the bathroom. I was occupied, using the greater part of my strength to hold down a raving madman until he finally succumbed to the drug and was taken away. Then I went to get Zelda. She said irritated, "I almost wet my pants waiting for you!" Other aides and nurses were available, but she likes me to be the one to lift her from chair to potty.

In the afternoon Patrick was found near death in his bed. His face was pushed deep into a pillow, and he was blue from the waist up from lack of oxygen. Two nurses spent a good hour bringing him around. Under normal circumstances Patrick is unable to move any extremity, so he probably suffered some kind of stroke that wrenched him into a difficult and airless position. Or, perhaps a careless aide just positioned him poorly.

Midge and Gracie came to a parting of the ways and are no longer roommates. They had a big fight, although just a few minutes later neither could remember it. Unfortunately, Gracie was entertaining family visitors at the time, and they complained about Midge's foul language. So Midge is out, relegated to a back hall.

My coworker Reba was suspended from work for five days. Apparently she let loose some insensitive remark to responsible family members. This new trouble adds financial strain to her already stormy life. In addition, it turns out that she recently discovered that she is pregnant. When the head nurse handed down her penalty, she asked Reba if she had anything to say in her defense. Reba said that she'd like to see some things changed, and then she proceeded to charge me with sexually harassing her by putting my hand on her shoulder. Later, Reba's husband called and added even more flavor to the mix, saying that I had visited them at home one day and touched Reba's leg.

The head nurse passed this along to me, as is her duty. As she was filling out an Employee Counseling form, she mumbled, "This is such a crock."

Reba said once that she thought I was "probably as rich as an old goat." So I speculate that she and her husband might be hoping for some kind of legal restitution. My first response was to hope that just ignoring this absurdity would be enough. Maybe this whole thing might drop of its own weight. I suggested that Reba and I be kept as far apart as possible.

Actually, it would be impossible to exaggerate my sexual disinterest in Reba. I am much more worried that I might never be interested in sex again after working here.

But I have certainly loved Reba's outlandish character, and even now I can't get very angry over this nonsense because I know that Reba has just been pouring her fears onto a convenient object (me), whom she correctly expects will roll over. Perhaps she is uncomfortable knowing that I do truly enjoy her remarkable nature, and she has no place to put me in her emotional repertoire.

The head nurse asked me to make a written response. This was my statement:

> I have read the above allegation, but I cannot say that I fully understand it. I do know that I have no control over another person's thinking. Vision is a product of what we are willing to see.
> I have worked beside this woman frequently and I have enjoyed (and suffered) her bravado and redoubtable flair for dominion. I relate to her as if she were an adolescent sister or

outlandish niece. It seems now, however, that she does not know what to do with my attitude.

I have twice told her in reply to her inquiries that I am not romantically interested in anyone who works here, that my aim is fixed on a certain woman in Japan whom I love for her delicate grace and sensitivity. The object of my desire is a willowy, almost frail lady and the most gentle creature I have ever known. I also stated my intention to return to Japan some day.

By contrast, the coworker in question is often comical in her gruff nature. I would not change anything about her. Still, it is impossible to exaggerate my disinterest in her as a sexual specimen. In fact, I find my experience working here to be diminishing to my libido. I have stated previously to her and others that a more real concern for me is whether or not I will ever be stirred by sexual desires again.

I did place my hand on her shoulder to get her attention. But how anyone can confuse this for a sexual signal or coercion is beyond me. I understand that her husband claims that I came to their trailer and touched her leg. That is a fabrication. The notion that I would go to their home and make a pass at her in the presence of her husband is just nuts. Nonetheless, I believe that she has too much goodness within her to swear to such a falsehood.

I understand that this friend of mine is under a great deal of pressure, financial and otherwise. To help relieve some stress I suggest that we put as much space between the two of us as is practical in the workplace. I might also suggest for her that the second shift is a great deal less stressful than days and that adjusting her schedule to evenings may provide some relief. At one point she has mentioned a desire to do just that.

It is a shame that this woman is willing to discard a perfectly decent friendship in her need to vent. I don't think she is malicious. I believe this allegation is a result of pressure. This came up as she was being suspended from work for misbehavior, a highly charged situation for anyone. Perhaps she is retreating, defending her boundaries of control by lashing out at someone who she believes will not retaliate. By diverting attention, blaming another, she protects herself. She has her own life to work out.

And I have mine. After I heard of this from the DON, it so disconcerted me that I went to Wal-Mart and bought a bread machine.

Reba failed to show up for work following her suspension, and her allegation against me was pretty much laughed off as "delusions of glamour." She also reported the nursing home to the Elderly Abuse Hotline for being understaffed.

We are, in fact, in the midst of a severe staff shortage and an accompanying crisis in morale. Our owner, who did not seem too upset about it, commented simply, "We go through staff."

One night recently five out of six scheduled aides failed to show up. A week ago, six new people were hired, and all but one quit after their two-day orientation.

I was called in again, the evening before my day off. We had only two aides on duty to care for 124 residents. When I arrived, Gina—all 105 pounds of her—was busting her hump caring for seventy-five helpless residents, some of whom outweighed her by over a hundred pounds. She was not complaining or acting beleaguered. On the contrary, she was into it, stoking like an Ironman competitor. At the same time I noticed that her charge nurse was seated at the nurse's station, enjoying a nice long personal phone call, apparently oblivious to the surrounding difficulties. A med tech, hanging out in the front office, was casually paging through a Christmas gift catalog. Gina's sole coworker was a novice aide who was so consumed with her fury at this unequal situation that she refused to move or talk. She sat immobilized and steaming, her glaring eyes burning a hole into the front nurses' station.

The following day another aide and I were left to feed twenty-seven helpless residents in the front dining hall while two office ladies found an empty dining table and proceeded to chat and have lunch. I suggested to them, since they are nice ladies, that they might like to help out in a pinch. I did not know how they could enjoy their visit while seated amid so many stolid people with plates of food gelling before their eyes. The ladies said that they could not help because they were not "licensed to help feed residents," and that they would not know what to do if someone started to choke. Oh well.

Ron is one of our best aides. He has decided that he's had enough, so he wrote out a note of resignation. I found his departure depressing, as he has dedication, a tender heart, and strong arms. I tried to talk him out of it. I approached the owner's wife, Daphne, and suggested that she might want to take a minute to try to turn him around. In the year that I have worked here, Ron is the only person I've ever heard actively defending our owners. But she said glibly, "Let him quit if he wants to." Oh well.

Then Beula's ex-husband died. It's true they'd lived on different halls, but after their twenty-six-year marriage ended, Beula and Bill remained good friends. Five days after his death, I expressed my sympathies to Beula, but she had no idea that Bill, her friend and ex-husband had died. At first she refused to believe me. I mentioned this to the lady in the front office who normally takes care of family relations. I thought that this was a simple lapse of attention, but she told me that since they were divorced, Bill's death was of no concern to Beula. Oh well.

So all week I have been hit with this question in various forms: How do we learn to care? Where does it start and when does it end? When is caring real? What kills compassion and what makes it thrive? Can we truly relieve suffering in others? I've seen myself get sensitive and then get caught up in my own stress to the point of becoming numb. I see how caring can nourish dependence as well as appreciation. I know that there is no end to suffering, no matter how pure our intentions, or how dedicated our acts. I cannot separate myself from these conundrums. I walk past residents who are begging me for help every day. I have no clear answer.

Tracy Kidder wrote a book, *Old Friends,* about life within a particularly fine nursing home. He quotes a resident: "The nurses and aides all have troubles. That's why they're so nice." Maybe difficulty assaults the ego and sensitizes us to the pains of others. Perhaps trials just give us the opportunity to become empathetic. After all, not all screw-ups are compassionate, but great pain can certainly help us step back a bit, which may be the beginning of understanding.

Allow me to ruminate on a thought from Thich Nhat Hanh, a Vietnamese monk. To paraphrase: Think of what pleases us in life as flowers, and what we don't want as garbage. In the West people try to keep just the flowers and throw out the garbage. In the East we love the flowers just as much, but we also hold great reverence for the garbage. By this act we transform it into good compost for the flowers.

The trick seems to be to embrace outrageous misfortune and respect it for what it can do for us. Garbage comes our way regardless. Fighting life's displeasures only solidifies our suffering. It's like wanting to have a magnet with only the positive pole.

In his book *Still Here,* Ram Das writes that we cannot transform an energy unless we bless it.

One of my favorite residents, Mimi, is undergoing some kind of change. She still hears ethereal music in the morning and mostly maintains her emotional composure. However, she is now subject to fitful spells of confusion and homesickness. She wanders the halls, standing before other residents' doorways studying the name plaques. She wants "to go to St. Joe's." She says, "I've got to go home and tend to my baby! What should I do?"

I am helpless to respond to her adequately. I'm told that according to our records she has never been married and has never had children. What ancient dramas may be replaying in her mind we will never know. My written messages to her on her whiteboard carry no discernible effect. She discards my responses with a brush of her hand. She simply reads them and repeats her questions and her demands. All I am able to do is use exaggerated hand motions to convey that she will have to stay put. I lamely offer her a small milkshake and move on to another task. Again my compassion ends in defeat. Again I am unable to take the pain away.

Charline, Ro's daughter, is upset with me. She came in this Sunday morning at 9:30 and found just two inches of water and no ice in her mother's carafe. Charline is quiet and sweet by nature, but she is worried about her mother's water intake. Ro's recent urinary tract infection may have been exacerbated by a need for greater amounts of fluid. So Charline stood in her mother's room, correctly stating that this is the fourth time in two weeks that she has found her mother without ice water. She said that she is going to call the owner on Monday morning. "I can only conclude that this is neglect," she said accusingly.

I stood in silence, taking her slings and arrows directly to my chest. I made no excuses nor disagreed with her in any way. Neither did I apologize. I know that Ro drinks prodigious amounts of water, and I know that she pees like a ruptured fire hose. So I privately doubt that Ro is dehydrated, but I mentioned none of this in our defense. I let our long-suspended silence hang in the air absorbing the blows of Charline's rightful concern for her mother.

By Tuesday we have a new policy in place. A nurse initials a form verifying that Ro's carafe is to be renewed with ice water by 7 A.M. (normally ice is passed by about 10 A.M.). By Friday, I notice that the new policy is already abandoned in the hectic pace of yet another confused morning. As usual, a new policy succumbs to its own cumbersome weight and staffing shortages. There are always new fires to put out.

The following week I was again called in to work on my day off. Even before I got to work I was short-tempered, resenting my loss of rest. I was mad at myself for agreeing to do what I want to get away from. The moment I clocked in, three hall lights lit up simultaneously. I was sent to clean up Ro's feces from her bed rails, sheet, floor, and fingernails. As it happened, her roommate, Marge, decided she had to go to the bathroom, and someone had parked her in her wheelchair outside the closed door to their room. Unknown to me as I began the big cleanup, Charline had also arrived. She stood by the door waiting to visit her mother. So from behind a closed door she heard me yell to Marge, "You don't want to come in here right now." And with clear frustration in my voice, I admonished Ro to "try to get it in the toilet next time. That's what the toilet is for." When I finally opened the door, Charline entered. She went out of her way to be kind to me. She even insisted on making Ro's bed. On my way out I grabbed the carafes and filled them with ice water.

Marge has missed her bath again. Last week I squeezed her in, in place of Ivy. More than most residents, Ivy will battle me in the shower, so I just traded her spot on the bath schedule for Marge's. That was last week.

Again this week the evening shift has been short; and Marge, who is no favorite with many, was left unwashed. So during the day, Marge asked me to summon the owner's wife, Daphne, for her. Shortly thereafter Daphne approached me and told me to be sure to give Marge a bath. "Do it today! I promised her. Fit it in."

I asked Daphne to select which other assigned task she wanted me to neglect in its place. I could have gone on to make the case more strongly, but there was no need. Daphne went to a co-worker, who readily agreed to bathe Marge later in the day.

The following morning Marge, with her clean hair, had me potty her three times before nine o'clock. This is a little much for me. She has every right to pee whenever she wants, but "lift and wipe" over and over again gets a little tiresome as a form of distraction. So I needled her, telling her with some exaggeration that she'd "gotten my ass in a grinder with the owner's wife." This put a worry in Marge's mind. Three times throughout the day she pulled me aside to assure me that she'd never said a word against me ". . . ever, and I'll hit anyone who does."

Walter and Bud were moved to the back hall, farther away from the front entrance. They are typical guys: crude as carnival barkers, sullen, drooling, and profane. The administration wants to protect the general public from the unpleasant sights of our workplace. It's good marketing practice to keep the front halls looking nice. That's primarily where visitors and prospective family members are taken for tours of the facility. Rooms toward the front are large, carpeted, and equipped with private shower units in the bathrooms. Toward the rear the rooms are smaller, simpler, and have tiled floors. It's time for Walter and Bud to get shipped to the back. Feeble, bedridden Harold thereby becomes our Lone Ranger, the sole representative of the male gender on 300 Hall. Three-quarters of the men are assigned to the back halls to drool and slump in solipsistic nirvana, dull haze, or sleep.

Meanwhile, demented women in flowery dresses wander along the front halls in aimless clutches. These groups remind me of ever-shifting schools of fish. No particular one of them decides where the group will turn next. It's as if they are guided by a shared consciousness, foraging the halls for scraps of family life, eluding and confusing the predatory male sharks that lurk about. Ladies misidentify each other, but they prefer that to being alone. Women clean up well by comparison with the men.

A new eighty-five-year-old lady was moved into Walter and Bud's room. Ada is clearheaded—not a thing wrong with her mind. But she is heavy set, and she hits the call button quite a lot. My first impression was, Here's another heavy complainer to deal with. But in just a couple of days I have begun to know her. Her complaint is real. Three weeks ago she broke her hip. The surgeon screwed a pin in her leg to repair it. Unfortunately, Ada's bones lack sufficient density to keep the screws in place, so pressure and movement keep dislodging the screws. Now one of the metal screws in particular is working its way deeper into the ball-and-socket joint every time she moves her leg. It sounds excruciating. The doctor surely has his own reasons for not wanting to extract this sharp and ragged edge, which digs and twists into her hip and causes considerable pain. If I were her, I'd look for another surgeon.

We have a somewhat similar case with a woman in the back. She had hip replacement surgery, but then her body rejected the implant. So the doctor removed the artificial hip and left her with nothing at all to stand on.

Staffing shortages continue. I notice that when I am left to care for twenty-seven residents alone, I am forced to take a lot of shortcuts. So I learn how to get away with minimal care. Once these shortcuts become part of my routine, they tend to stay put. I do not unlearn them; by nature, shortcuts are easier and quicker. I am reaching limits in my motivation to care. What is happening to my loving compassion? A resentful side of me is coming out.

I see my patience and gentleness running thin. I am less tolerant of Marty's incessant plaint, "To-o-omm, does my son still live at Indian Lake?" So now I treat Marty in a less condescending fashion. Yes, her condition is pitiful, but under this endless grind, I see no reason to enslave myself to her indulgences. What good is it to constantly reassure her of facts that she already knows perfectly well? Am I not reinforcing her emotional weakness?

I declared an end: no more caving in to her constant calls for attention and reassurance. Now I grow numb to her wailing. I put her on the toilet one morning, but she could not produce shit. I told her that I would have to leave her there. Knowing that this would start her crying, I said, "I've got to go. You might as well start your air-raid-siren wailing now." And guess what, she held her peace. It worked, but what am I turning into? A burnout?

Zelda now lets me potty her more quickly and directly. I put her on the john and run out the door. No problem.

Marge, on the other hand, will happily cut off her nose to spite her face. She went home for a birthday celebration at her sister's house. I loaded her in the car and put her wheelchair in the front office. When Marge got back that evening, the front office was locked, leaving her wheelchair out of reach. She had to borrow another. Her family went ballistic and even called the state with their complaint. Marge was furious with me, "You'll never get anything to eat from me, ever!"

I claimed to be human and slumped off with a shrug. Shortly thereafter all was forgotten and she offered me a yet another fruit pie.

As it happened, the state inspectors did show up. They'd heard too many complaints and knew that we had a growing number of bedsores generated in-house. So, for an entire week, the state inspectors stood in the halls holding clipboards, probing into our routines. I exchanged greetings with one of them as he was making notes on some physical changes that were needed on a fire wall. I told him that the owners were going to squawk about the cost he was imposing on them. I was startled to hear him respond: "I don't give a shit what they do. You have no idea what kind of lifestyle these people are accustomed to."

Marge had the gall to tell the inspectors every time she wanted to go to the bathroom, have a drink of ice water, take another shower.

"Well, I guess there's nobody to take me to the toilet," she'd announce loudly and a bit too dramatically. Suspecting abuse of power, I put a hat (a plastic container used to measure urine output) under her toilet seat. Marge told me to get it out of there, but I defied her. She didn't pee enough to cover the bottom of it. Marge gets her way, but I feel no affection for her today. Not every need is equally urgent, I decide.

In the early morning, as it happened, Marge and Marty and two others simultaneously demanded that I get them up. At 5 A.M. in the middle of 300 Hall, I blurt out in a stentorian voice, "Somebody's just going to have to have a little self-discipline around here!" A kindhearted little nurse was walking toward me at that moment. I saw her mouth drop open.

This precipitous change in me was long in coming. From the very beginning it had been impressed upon me that call lights are to be answered promptly. Resident requests are taken seriously. Old people are delicate and helpless. Their wish is our command.

But exhaustion is bringing up a different sense of balance. Maybe if I treat these people like responsible adults, they may begin to treat us a bit more reasonably and maybe respect themselves a tiny bit more in the process. I've come to realize that by indulging my residents I am not showing respect for them, nor for myself.

Marge skipped her after-breakfast potty time, I am sure as a special consideration for me. Then she went fishing for a compliment, "Tom, have I been to the bathroom today yet?" insisting I take notice.

"I don't know," I lied, not giving her an inch of concession.

With Marty, I started counting aloud the number of times she asked me, "Does my son still live at Indian Lake?" instead of answering her directly. (The first question of the day I gave away as a freebie.) By the time I wheeled her into breakfast I said, "That's four times."

Marty, visibly irritated, barked back, "Well, so what?"

"Because it's boring. It's annoying." I barked back.

So now Marty, instead of asking me about her son, asks for a drink of ice water when I pass within earshot. I comply, but not necessarily with my same old Johnny-on-the-spot eagerness.

"What's tomorrow?" she asked.

"Another day," I replied.

"Is Bert coming tomorrow?"

"Why can't you be happy today?"

"Because you're here and he's not," Marty retorted. Then she extended her arm toward me, a faint smile across her lips. I smile despite myself.

I still make a point of holding one-on-one conversations with Marty at least once a day to counterbalance my weary approach. Perhaps by default, our conversations turn to new subjects. Instead of doting on her, feeding her need for constant reassurance, we just chat. I read up on jokes for her. Our conversations become slightly more normal, one adult to another.

Zelda has been consciously restraining her requests. My appreciation for her rises. On my break I visit with her. She is my friend again.

And when I see a call light on, instead of dropping everything and rushing to the rescue, I make a mental note, "Oh, so-and-so probably has to go to the toilet. I'll get to that next."

Tinker got sick and died. I visited her in the hospital two days before she passed. She suffered far too much. I remember putting her tiny hand in my palm. It looked so delicate, not really human, and so light that I could not detect its weight. Our eyes met, but she was too weak to talk. Emotions ran strong in me, but I didn't say much. Oddly, her troublesome sister, Jamie, who worried about Tinker to the point of distraction, seemed immediately relieved. Her burden of responsibility lifted, Jamie is much more pleasant to be with lately.

Just after I clocked out, the other day, I saw a brand-new aide, a kind middle-aged woman, wide-eyed and attentive, bending over Marty. With the sweetest adoring tone she asked Marty if there was anything at all that she could do for her. Her words came out as melodious as baby talk. Marty was soaking up the fawning attention.

As I walked out the door I shook my head slightly and let out some air with a *pfff*. Then, taken aback by my own reaction, "Oh, my God, how sour have I become?"

I am full up with this place. I feel shamed and jaded. Today the nursing home seems like a colony of whiners: good people made petty by years of politely ignoring real but subtle needs of the heart.

Walter died on a quiet Wednesday afternoon. He had been in a gradual decline for months, but portions of his colorful style still flared up, even in the way he summoned our help, waving his one good hand as if he were orchestrating a legion of underlings. I could not help loving him. On Tuesday he started leaning heavily to the right in his wheelchair, no longer able to feed himself or hold himself upright. Even so, he still carried an air of dignity. Bent severely at the waist, he might have been a great cavalry officer wounded in battle and refusing to dismount his charger.

By the following morning, his focus started to dull and his skin tone became bluish and mottled. He entered unknown territory, becoming uncharacteristically frightened as he approached the threshold. To our credit, and to Walter's great comfort, a lovely young aide was allowed to stay with him for his final hours, holding his hand and stroking his brow.

Walter just faded away. I was there at the end, but I could not identify the exact moment when he left. His breaths became slower and were spaced further and further apart. Finally we realized there would be no more. Death itself must have been easy for him.

Moments later a Bible preacher, a strikingly handsome young man, came into the room. He knelt on one knee by Walter's bed. In a voice loud enough to traverse the entire space between heaven and hell, he began—although Walter was already gone at this point: "Walter, I want to read to you from the Holy Scriptures so you may repent your sins and accept Jesus as your Lord and personal Savior before you stand in His judgment." And he went on and on about how God would tell him, "I don't know you" if Walter didn't believe or do something just so. I got pretty irritated at this sincere young man, ministering to his first death, utterly out of sync and oblivious to all but his own agenda and rigid beliefs. Walter still had an oxygen line tucked under his nose, and the concentrator was still producing a mechanical rattle. The preacher said, "Walter, I know you may find this difficult right now, but the Bible says 'Sing unto the Lord His praises.'" I reached over and closed Walter's eyelids and then switched off the concentrator, hoping the young preacher would get the hint.

Finally he left, and the aide and I shared a quiet, sorrowful hug and repositioned Walter's body. We quietly recovered the sense of grief and dignity of the moment.

Back at the nurse's station, an LPN was saying, "Well at least Walter had his final consolation from the preacher. I'm sure it meant a lot to him." The aide and I let that go by. Later we concluded that the experience was probably important to the young preacher.

Walter had a handful of snapshots in the top drawer of his dresser, pictures from his farm in Minnesota. I kept a 3 x 5 photo of horses feeding in the snow as a remembrance of him.

Lola died unexpectedly. She had been sick for a few days with vomiting and diarrhea, but we thought that had cleared up.

I saw her at lunch on a Tuesday pulling herself through a maze of wheelchairs in the dining room. As usual, Lola was not talking or interacting with anyone. I moved her out of my way without bothering to excuse myself, as I was helping another resident beat a path to the toilet.

Lola was put to bed shortly after supper that evening, and at 9:30 they found her dead in her bed. She may have choked on her own vomit—they found a small spot of it dried on her sheets. We'll never know, though, because no autopsy was ordered. The state was assigned as Lola's guardian and quietly disposed of the body.

Though her son had paid no heed, Lola clung to the memory of Chas as her one source of pride and solace. She often threatened to report our behavior to him when our interventions disrupted her despair. As her only relative, Chas served as her legal guardian for awhile, but he later changed his phone to an unlisted number. Because we had lost all means of notifying him of her death, we had no place to send her personal belongings. So her sweatshirts and pants went to the laundry.

I packed up her remaining personal possessions. All that she owned was a tattered vinyl suitcase, a string of fake pearls, a magnifying glass, and two studio photos of her son. Her suitcase stayed up front in the social services office for a few weeks until someone decided that since Lola had left an outstanding debt with us, we probably would never locate Chas. We tossed the old suitcase in the dumpster.

A week later the son appeared to claim Lola's personal effects. He said he owes us nothing, and in fact, he thinks we owe him money! He also claims that his mother came in with an expensive gold watch. And he wanted it back. His disposition is surly and suspicious. I see that Lola left more unwieldy baggage behind than just an old suitcase.

Epilogue

Death plucks my ears and says, "Live—I am coming."
—Virgil

Some months ago I was asked about this book, about how it ends. My response was that it stops but it doesn't end. I draw no grand conclusions. I have no serious proposals for repairing our nursing homes.

I've just written down what happens here. I stuffed scraps of paper in the pocket of my scrub top and collected quotes and tidbits one at a time. My notes tended to ramble in circles just as some of our ambulatory residents do. The same sad observations come up time and again. It's like staring at a prison wall but in a slightly new light each day. I am like "All-timers": the mundane surprises me with renewed depth and texture. If I were a totally faithful writer, this project would end in bits and scraps, some half-words, and then perhaps a lot of blank space.

I see unbearable misfortunes right here in my own little town. In the beginning I saw these people as human aliens, a sweet harmless subspecies. But now I feel their sad seeds sprouting within me. I know that I am becoming one of these odd beings I lift and roll and wipe every day. What will I do when my turn comes up? Lash out like Marty? Manipulate staff like Zelda? Die unnoticed like Enoch?

Few of us are prepared for what happens. First we grow up and get stronger by the day. Then one day the process reverses. At first we deny and resist, but eventually we all surrender.

Working as an aide has certainly put its mark on me. I'm more aware now of what may lie ahead for me and for you. I can see how my body will creak and get uncool and rot. I may well get confused, depressed beyond all measure. I may wet my pants and not care. I've seen what time and loneliness do to a body, but none of this predicts where the heart will be.

Perhaps nursing homes in America are the product of our rugged individualism. We are the victims of our own indulgence and selfish freedom. Nursing homes are the outcome of our dreams of owning rather than belonging. Maybe we've no time for our parents (and ourselves) because we're too busy going after some thing we don't yet own. Nursing homes teach us that the price of freedom is separation.

Traditionally Buddhist monks began their training in the charnel grounds, meditating among decomposing corpses. The idea is to deeply internalize the entire cycle of life, to see ourselves as part of nature rather than as being apart. Here in North America, media and advertising would have us all pretend we are eternal teenagers.

I understand some readers find this book depressing. This is not a problem. It is the natural response as our minds struggle to accept the unacceptable. But running away, mentally fighting the idea, denial: these only prolong the difficulty. Suffering is the effect of wanting things to be different from how they truly are. Sooner or later we will give in to nature; we have no choice. Better to adjust sooner and become comfortable with our place in a greater life cycle. We can stop fighting our own nature.

It is a paradox, and a most difficult idea to convey: Once we

truly accept our mortality, the capacity for joy expands expo-
nentially. I at least am convinced that there is far more to us than
what is destined for the grave.

Especially as Americans, we know ourselves as unique individuals. But we are also part of the system we call "nature."

Imagine a single drop of water (this drop of water is special,
for it knows itself) in the ocean riding on the crest of a wave. Perhaps it knows the surface tension that separates it from all other
drops. But more likely it feels the power of the entire wave along
with all the other water droplets. It does not resist the wave; it
goes along for the ride. It does not pretend, "I am a huge drop
of water." It might say, "I am an integral part of this swell moving ever faster toward the shore." In the same way, when we recognize that we are not only unique but also part of a very large
system of laws, we can participate in the beauty and power of
nature's momentum.

Underdeveloped countries appear to deal better with old age,
perhaps because economically they have no choice. Their practice is to allow death rather than to fight it off at astronomical
costs. As a result everyone is assured that there is a time and place
for every human experience, that everyone has a part to play, and
that everyone belongs somewhere. Here, more often we belong
to the mortgage company, the IRS, the BMW.

I have become a different kind of person after working in long-
term care.

People enter a nursing home with varying expectations. Many
come expecting to die. And a few do die in very short order,
within days or even hours, but most who wish for death fail to
get God's immediate cooperation. Some seem condemned to stay
alive until they learn to like it here. Eventually residents find that
their life goes on inside a nursing home pretty much as it did before. Except that within more help is available. They may even
find new friendships and interests that they would never have

considered while holed up alone, perhaps in a tiny rent-subsidized apartment.

Some come expecting us to wait on them hand and foot. They imagine they will receive the one-on-one care, the constant attention, that only the wealthy can afford. At home, if someone has an accident, you just clean it up, but what happens in a facility if five people get diarrhea at the same time? Disappointments are bound to arise.

Some families don't care what we do with dear Mom, just as long as it doesn't cost the family anything beyond what Medicaid picks up. So many families live in a constant state of civil war; so many children and parents disown each other. Tragically, many parents or children die before family rifts are repaired.

Most neophytes expect our Alzheimer's wing to be a padded jail. The exit lock is coded to protect residents from wandering off, but soon after their loved ones move in, families typically find it's refreshing to see geriatrics acting together like toddlers, not even noticing who's male and who's female. Something magical seems to happen when Alzheimer's patients mix exclusively with each other. They get lost in a moment that has no name. They communicate in some primal way and settle into a language of tone, cadence, and emotion. Our Alzheimer's wing is by far the happiest hall in the building.

I've often seen offspring and parent play the guilt card against each other, as children reluctantly become their parents' providers. Residents will malign our care, complaining to their children in exaggerated terms, hoping to extort a return passage back home if they paint a black enough picture of long-term care.

"My children deceived me" and "Them damned kids stole my house" are also familiar refrains. In general, accusations run harshest against the family members who have served the longest and care the most. The real complaint is that no one can turn back the clock and restore the ability to run and play outside. I have learned that loving offspring often make the worst judges of their parents' capabilities.

Often clients are quite pleased with us for long periods. And then when dementia takes a precipitous toll, leaving the aged one mute and locked in a fetal position with their skin breaking down, family members may need someone to blame. When doctors overmedicate a patient, the family might target the nursing home for "drugging Mom to make your job easier." When pharmaceutical companies make scandalous profits on their expensive drugs—and they do—families suspect that it is the nursing home that is ripping them off.

To my amazement, I have seen how it's possible to become aged without maturing, to live out an entire life without ever achieving adulthood. As long as those around us support our neuroses, we will take the path of least resistance and find no need to grow. I've seen sweet old ladies die remaining fierce bigots or spoiled brats to the very end. I know that in the outside world there is an unwritten law about people in wheelchairs with gray hair: we are all supposed to fawn over how sweet and cute they are. But that's oversimplified and ultimately demeaning. One eighty-five-year-old I know will stomp her feet and throw a tantrum, crying, "But I want it" until she gets whatever she is demanding. She has not yet truly learned that others coexist in her world.

One evening this woman stood in the front hall and tearfully insisted on having five bananas. The grocery truck was behind schedule that week; there were only eight bananas in the entire facility with 115 residents. They would be needed for breakfast in the morning, and Parkinson's patients have bananas prescribed for their potassium value. Yet this woman got all but three. The following day I asked her daughter-in-law, "How did she manage to live this long without getting strangled?" She said, "It was always just easier to give in to her."

The DON heard about my question and made me give her family a houseplant.

Nursing homes house the unbeautiful side of life. This is the hard reality—pretense and false hope fall away at our doorstep. Most people do the best they can in difficult situations. That applies to residents and staff alike. When I think of what they do, day in and day out, I am very proud of my coworkers. In just a short period I've seen how rapidly time assaults the body as we approach our personal finish line. From the outside it may appear that nothing is happening, but the body's clock is racing at an ever accelerating speed. So often I see those who take the easiest path regret it later. They settle into a wheelchair because it's easier. Soon it's too late to stand up without assistance. Then just when all hope is lost, they suddenly wish with all their heart that they could dance the jig just one more time.

I also see others who stay full of spunk and humor right up to the end. Many of our residents are quite contented to live with wonderful memories. I am amazed at how many residents have the fortitude and balance to accept decrepitude with grace and good humor. They manage to keep the heart open as the body shuts down. How well we approach our own death tells the world what kind of person we grew with our life.

I have been astonished at how well our facility continues to operate despite all the gruesome realities and miserable shortcomings we face every day.

But I also wonder what would happen if we dropped our feigned hope that we can indefinitely forestall the inevitable. What if instead we really concentrated on honoring the lives entrusted to us, making them as comfortable and respected as possible? What if we thought of this place as a gathering of life patterns and outcomes, a showcase for honesty and repression, a foster home for the inner child within us to the very end?

The constant unrelenting ache of loneliness in this place certainly illustrates how much families really mean to us. What if a proud and peaceful death here was a crowning achievement rather than a failure of medicine? We hide death as if we are ashamed of it: "Lost another one." When a resident dies here, we lock down the hall and hide the news and the body from fellow residents, as if they were unable to handle the one reality that clearly permeates these halls.

I visited a TB sanitarium in the Far East one time. A small girl, about four years old, had just died in the dormitory. A good nun there stroked the little body tenderly. The girl's playmates stood close by, taking in the scene. Their demeanor was serious and quiet, but composed. After a few minutes they simply went off a few feet away and resumed their routine business, playing quietly.

A few miles up the highway from this nursing home the Humane Society takes in a constant stream of puppies and kittens. As in any such place you can hear the dogs yelping, pack animals complaining about being separated from their social nature. They only want to belong. It's in their bones. In the same way, belonging is in our bones too. Why can we not structure this simple truth into long-term care?

Occasionally someone brings a puppy into our nursing home and the results are generally wonderful. I have seen puppies sleep peacefully for hours in the laps of residents who are normally restless. Demented or sane, the residents often beam with joy at having a love object to hold and cuddle. The animals seem to adjust their behavior to suit the needs of the residents. Some of our residents object, but these are not the open hearts among us.

What would it take to meld these two types of lonely hearts to create joy and caring and belonging for both? We could have animals available (the so-called Eden Alternative). It would cost more, but would the cost still be too high if *we* were the residents? Could a nursing home somehow be a touch point for emotionally abandoned or molested children? Would we dare let a lost orphan curl up on an old lap just as we let a puppy do? Perhaps we could even simulate a real community. These are not new ideas. They are also troublesome and inconvenient, as well as expensive. Yes, they would cut into the profit margin. But why is it necessary to profit from the infirm? I know these may seem like pipe dreams, but at least we could lean in this direction. It takes so little to touch a lonely heart.

At present nursing homes are designed more like outmoded zoos. Residents are kept in small rooms, emotionally isolated. Occasionally they are visited by family members who reach through the bars and offer them treats. We keep their bodies clean and presentable. We truly forget that the boundaries of our nature far exceed the limits of our skin. We invest huge amounts of money to maintain the body while leaving the person to languish, cut off from all they love.

What would elder care look like if, from its inception, it was not about controlling costs and maximizing profits? What if it really was about our basic need to be meaningful and connected, right up to the end? What would happen if we kept infirm people in the realm of "normal" life? Is it possible that we are robbing ourselves and our children of a primal lesson: how to age and how to die? I firmly believe that both the young and the old would profit from the mix. By witnessing my own mother's decline and death, I saw how one can die with grace and dignity. How can such a lesson be measured?

What if, instead of forbidding employees to bring their children to work as we presently do, we provided a day-care satellite area that encouraged kids to come and stay, to mix and mingle. Perhaps some minors and residents might "adopt" each other if grandma is not tucked away in a corner. What if residents had the opportunity to teach some living history? Or to read, act lovingly, act goofy? When I was a child, I loved it when a grandparent took me aside to teach me something—I felt safe; I got personal attention. But at the same time I hated school. What if residents made a little money tending latchkey kids? Well, there would be minimum-wage requirements, OSHA concerns, FICA . . .

We are social by nature, yet here we are, isolating, segregating, and separating, all the while incurring a hidden cost with our antiseptic approach. By taking away all responsibilities and duties from residents, we contribute to their despair. When a resident throws a tantrum, we offer pacifying sweets to be eaten alone.

About compassion, I have concluded that it does not imply meeting every demand and request put upon you. Neither does it suggest ignoring the needy or leaving them to fend for themselves. Compassion does not need to feed neuroses and indulgences.

This is how I have come to feel both softened and jaded. But would I feel this way if I had more time with the people I became attached to? I was a different person when I wasn't chronically exhausted, when I had sufficient time off to recharge myself, when I took enough time to protect my own health. I do not like the person I became under pressure. I was not the man I want to be. Originally I tried to leave my own feelings and needs out of the equation, and just give. But this tack cannot last.

There are dilemmas involved in the context of all caregiving work—whether you are the parent of a child with attention deficit/hyperactivity disorder or an aide caring for an incontinent ninety-four-year-old. Human vulnerability and dependence create relentless demands. But that relentlessness was tolerable when I first came to work here. I had more to give when I was better rested, when I worked beside other aides, when I had days off, time to tend to myself. I deteriorated when I had less sleep and respite. I forgot to respect myself.

There is a lesson here. Taking care of the sick and old is inherently taxing. When you deprive aides of respect and reward, it becomes an unbearable, soul-degrading burden. I failed to create compassion when I forgot to respect myself. That key, self-respect, has become a new beacon. Lesson learned.

Exhausting oneself at the behest of others breeds resentment, not compassion. I've come to think that what matters is more a matter of style and motive, of how a task is done, and what is intended by it. It is about opening the self to another's inner life.

Compassion breeds more compassion. A small group of heroic family members come here every day. They visit spouses or parents who are often severely demented, totally unable to respond to any social input; nonetheless, these steadfast few seem consistently happy, contented souls. I see them hobble in on canes, or visit after a long day at work, or drive up in ancient cars, or in at least one case in a brand new Cadillac. These transcendent souls refuse to forget the love of years gone by. You can see it in their faces. Their loyalty and filial piety somehow propel them far beyond the apparently tragic circumstance of the moment. Obviously these folks have traveled a long emotional road; they have somehow come full circle to arrive at true contentment and altruism. This is magic. I see these few wonderful souls as a powerful spiritual force that permeates the air in ways both subtle and profound yet rarely recognized. I believe that they influence the ambiance of these halls in an almost sacred way. Day after day, they remind us all of what this place really could be.

I now take serious note of the effects of burnout and exhaustion on my own spirit. Previously I would have thought it callous to just walk on, ignoring a sweet old lady who was pleading to me for help. Privately I had criticized social workers for being aloof and maintaining a professional, hands-off distance. Now I see how we can only respond to the most pressing demands of our residents.

I wheeled Marge to the dining hall for supper as I was about to leave after a long day at work. As usual, in her boredom and impatience she asked to be taken to her table a full half-hour early. That evening she put me in a playful mood. I knelt by her side and placed my elbow on her wheelchair armrest. We feigned an arm wrestling match. She grimaced dramatically and acted as if she was biting my wrist in order to gain the upper hand.

I yielded and we laughed. Then our eyes locked for just a second. We looked deeply into each other, smiling, acknowledging real friendship.

I pulled her up to her table. She asked for buttermilk. I hoofed my way to the kitchen to relay her message to the staff. The night cook said, "No, if we give her buttermilk now she won't eat any of her supper." So rather than deliver the unwanted news back to Marge, and put up with her barking, I just sneaked out through the kitchen.

Three hours later she was dead of a heart attack.

When I heard the news, my initial reaction was, My God, why didn't I just get her a glass of buttermilk? But it's unlikely that her life would have ended significantly happier.

It also reminded me that whenever you say good-bye, you never know if you will see that person alive again.

Compassion respects the adult as an adult, as well as comforting the vulnerable parts within a wounded soul. Compassion also shows equal respect for the doer; we must have compassion for ourselves in equal measure. We must attune to our own sorrows before we can fully attend to another's. Compassion is both intimate and respectful, easing pain while honoring our commonality.

I do not know precisely what compassion is. It cannot be dissected without sounding identical to love, or wholeness or understanding. But there were moments when I served as a kind of key that unlocked a resident's mood, and then for a moment we both felt free. By doing this repeatedly, certain strictures within my own psychology relaxed. I learned that I have an intrinsic value to people who had never before met me. These feeble strangers taught me a nonspecific kind of loving, which in turn informed me that what I do matters to the world.

Long-term care offered me a long and fruitful meditation on how we meet our end. It's about how our bodies fall apart. Religious traditions around the globe have advocated that we look directly at the impermanence of our lives. Medieval Christian monks kept skulls in their cells to meditate on death: powerful memento mori. Buddhist monks meditate on corpses. These practices grow not out of morbid fascination but out of a paradoxical pursuit of vitality. When I fully realize that I am going to die, the current moment takes on a preciousness that had been taken for granted before.

"You jump into the fire and come out in the water," says Ram Das.

Only through a fearless comprehension of our own mortality can we achieve a clear view of reality. In the profound realization that we cannot hold on to health, nor to possessions, nor to relationships, comes spiritual maturity. Then we are likely to fully appreciate what we so easily take for granted—our health, our family, this very moment. To see the commonplace with renewed freshness is to be born again. This is the same phenomenon reported by people who have faced death through major illness or accident or so-called near-death experiences. Priorities change. Superficialities drop away.

One day we will all lose our health. It can be a blessing to be able to see the end coming. It gives everyone time to adjust. Those who can navigate infirmity with grace are admirable; those who remain undefeated transcend the need for anyone else's opinion.

Every one of us humans is pointed in the same direction. We can put the inevitable out of our mind for awhile, but it will catch up one day, guaranteed. In fact, death is the only guarantee we have been granted by life. Yet most of us pretend we will be the only one to escape it.

I try to imagine myself in a geriatric body, living in a nursing home. I expect that I'll handle it well. Funny, though. I can never quite capture a clear image of what I will be like. There are so many possible ways to go.

About the Author

Tom Gass has divided his life between working in the
trades and using his psychology degree in a variety of social work settings—as director of a half-way house, Head
Start teacher on an Indian reservation, and director of a
group home for developmentally disabled adults. At the
age of thirteen he entered a Catholic seminary, which
included a year of silence. At a meditation enclave he prac-
ticed deliberate, reflective awareness, a discipline he expanded in each of the twenty-three countries in which he
has lived and performed various volunteer activities. When
his mother became ill with cancer he returned from a decade in Asia to help her through the process of dying. That
experience inspired his decision to work in long term care,
as chronicled in this book, first as a nurse's aide and eventually as director of social services. He currently lives in
the Midwest.

About the Writer of the Foreword

Bruce C. Vladeck is Professor of Health Policy and
Geriatrics at Mount Sinai School of Medicine in New
York City. He has been involved in long-term care for
more than twenty-five years, as the author of *Unloving*

Care: The Nursing Home Tragedy (1980), a member of the Committee on Nursing Home Regularion of the Institute of Medicine of the National Academy of Sciences, Administrator of the Health Care Financing Administration (the federal agency responsible for Medicare and Medicaid) from 1993 through 1997, and the Director of a national nursing home company, among many other activities.

About the Series Editors

Suzanne Gordon is an award-winning journalist whose work focuses on the health care workforce, political culture, and women's issues. She is the author of five books, including *Life Support: Three Nurses on the Front Lines,* and coauthor of *From Silence to Voice: What Nurses Know and Must Communicate to the Public.* **Sioban Nelson** is Associate Professor at the School of Nursing, The University of Melbourne, Australia. A registered nurse and a nursing historian, she has written extensively on the history of health, ethics, and health policy.